Stan

SERGEI TCHERKASSKI

Stanislavsky and Yoga

Translated from Russian by
VRENELI FARBER

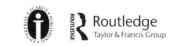

Holstebro – Malta – Wrocław
London – New York
2016

ICARUS Publishing Enterprise is a joint initiative
of Odin Teatret (Denmark), the Grotowski Institute (Poland)
and Theatre Arts Researching the Foundations (Malta)

Cover design Barbara Kaczmarek
Typesetting Tadeusz Zarych
Index Agata Kaczmarek

Published by
Icarus Publishing Enterprise and Routledge
www.icaruspublishing.com
www.routledge.com

The Grotowski Institute
Rynek-Ratusz 27, 50-101 Wrocław, Poland

Routledge
2 Park Square, Milton Park, Abingdon, OX14 4RN, UK
711 Third Avenue, New York, NY 10017, USA
Routledge is an imprint of Taylor and Francis Group, an informa business

ISBN 978-1-138-69178-0 (paperback)
ISBN 978-1-138-69177-3 (hardback)

Printed in Poland by JAKS

Contents

Foreword

More than a hundred years have passed since Stanislavsky realized that the creation of a 'grammar of dramatic art',[1] which gradually became the main occupation of his life, cannot be reduced to a collection of 'advice to players' of the sort that Shakespeare, Diderot, and Lessing before him had successfully given. It was necessary to attempt to systematize the *rules of nature* in the creative work of an actor, to find a *system* for the elements of the actor's sense of self. Thus was born the term *System* in Stanislavsky's manuscript written in June 1909.[2] Three pages from Stanislavsky's notebook, preserved in the museum of the Moscow Art Theatre, expound sequentially the basic elements of the System. (The pencil-written pages are very legible even after a hundred years; this suggests that, ironically, not many have wished to look at this unpublished document.)

The System remained in the hands of its creator for the first thirty years of its existence, during which time it developed and was modified so dramatically that today many think that it is necessary to contrast the early and late Stanislavsky, and they consider his discoveries of the 1930s as the essence of the System. In so doing, the very concept of 'early' Stanislavsky unavoidably acquires an evaluative character and becomes a synonym for 'immature'. It is as if the early period of the System (the 1910s) is negated by the late period (the 1930s);

[1] 'Some sort of grammar of dramatic art haunts me, some sort of book of preparatory practical exercises', wrote Stanislavsky in a letter to Vera Pushkareva-Kotliarevskaya on 20 June 1902. See K. S. Stanislavskii, *Sobranie sochinenii* (Collected Works), 9 vols (Moscow: Iskusstvo, 1988–99), II (1989), 498–99 (hereafter referred to as Stanislavskii, *Ss* 9).

[2] The term 'system' first appeared in Stanislavsky's work 'Programme of the Article: My System', written in June 1909 (unpublished document from the Archive of the Museum of the Moscow Art Theatre, K. S. Stanislavsky Collection, no. 628, pp. 46–48). Though Stanislavsky himself, and other authors wrote the word 'system' differently (the 'system', the System, or simply the system), («система», Система, или просто система), in the present book this term is written in accordance with the norms of contemporary language – the *Stanislavsky System* or the *System*.

it is unavoidably condescending towards the first steps or the first efforts. Ideological attitudes, according to which only in the Soviet era was Stanislavsky able to overcome his 'delusions' of the 1910s, also played a role. Soviet scholarship held that these delusions were the result of the influence of 'bourgeois science' and 'idealistic philosophy'.

In 1991, Anatoly Smeliansky, publishing the second volume of a new collection of works by Stanislavsky, wrote:

> Until the present time it was impossible to consider the question of the correlation of the System and the 'Method of Physical Actions' as resolved.[3] There is a view according to which 'the method of physical actions' is not an addition to what Stanislavsky did before the beginning of the 1930s, but a qualitative change in his conceptions of the nature of the actor's and director's creative work. An alternative view is one that takes into account the deep connection of Stanislavsky's last experiments with the spirit of the System and with the search for both indirect paths to and new 'lures' in the organic creative work of the actor.[4]

Two decades have passed but in the consciousness of theatrical practitioners there is no single, unequivocal, interpretation of the problem described above. The reason for this is patently simple: there are too few scholarly and systematic works devoted to the early period of the development of the System and to those fundamental explorations of the laws of the actor's craft which were undertaken by Stanislavsky in the 1910s. This cannot fail to be surprising if one compares the lists of students of the early and late periods of the System, namely the students of

[3] For Smeliansky, the term 'Method of Physical Actions' means the totality of discoveries by Stanislavsky in the 1930s, both the Method of Psycho-Physical Actions and the Method of Action Analysis. The technically correct and more helpful English translation of the Russian term *metod deistvennogo analiza* is 'the Method of Analysis through Action', also known as 'Analysis through Action'. In English, this method is commonly called Action Analysis or Active Analysis. This book will use Action Analysis and Analysis through Action interchangeably.

[4] A. M Smeliansky, 'Professiia – artist' in Stanislavskii, Ss 9, II (1989), 29.

Stanislavsky in the First Studio of the Moscow Art Theatre and those in the Opera-Dramatic Studio. In the First Studio the lessons of Stanislavsky and Sulerzhitsky were assimilated by Evgeny Vakhtangov, Michael Chekhov, Boris Sushkevich, Richard Boleslavsky, Alexei Popov, Sofia Giatsintova, Maria Ouspenskaya, Serafima Birman, Alexei Dikii, Illarion Pevtsov, Vladimir Gotovtsev, Valentin Smyshliaev, Vera Soloviova, Andrius Jilinsky, Maria Durasova, and Alexander Cheban. In a word, a whole pleiad of the most well-known masters of the Russian and, indeed, the world stage was born here. And who, other than specialists, remembers the names of the students of the Opera-Dramatic Studio? Moreover, many of Stanislavsky's early students proved to be receptive to his later ideas (Alexei Popov became one of the leading specialists on the Method of Action Analysis; Richard Boleslavsky, having started with the fundamentals gained in the First Studio, independently came to many of the ideas of Stanislavsky of the 1930s), while his later students at times were deaf to his early experiments (a sad example is Mikhail Kedrov).

In my earlier studies,[5] I have already argued with the oversimplified model which has taken root in the minds of many theatrical practitioners, that there is an early Stanislavsky (with affective memory as the leading element of the System) and there is a late Stanislavsky (with action as the leading element of the System), and that the late period cancels the early one. Research reveals a constant presence in the System of ideas and elements which are traditionally linked only with the initial period of its development. This allows one to formulate a new appreciation of the early period of development of the System, understood as a 'whole entity'.

[5]   S. D. Tcherkasski, 'The Directing and Teaching of Richard Boleslavsky and Lee Strasberg as an Experiment in the Stanislavsky System's Development' (D.Sc. dissertation in Theatre Studies, Saint Petersburg State Theatre Arts Academy, 2012). An English language synopsis is published in the article: Sergei Tcherkasski, 'The System Becomes the Method: Stanislavsky – Boleslavsky – Strasberg', *Stanislavski Studies*, e-journal, 3 (2013), 92–138 <http://stanislavskistudies.org>.

And it allows one to draw the conclusion that the early period in its essence is a *basic* period, a component, not a cancelled part of the System and of the modern methodology of an actor's creative work.[6] The importance of this conclusion for contemporary actor training seems so significant that it is fitting to proclaim the slogan: 'Forward to the early Stanislavsky!'

A detailed study of the early period of the development of the Stanislavsky System is still waiting to be carried out, both in archives and in practical rehearsals. It is necessary to examine the work of Alexander Adashev's Studio (the practice of the Stanislavsky System before the Stanislavsky System, so to speak) and to concentrate on the pedagogy (namely the pedagogical process, and not the history of productions and their artistic analysis) of the First Studio of the Moscow Art Theatre. Most important is to look closely at the lessons of Richard Boleslavsky and Maria Ouspenskaya in the American Laboratory Theatre and at the actor training established by Lee Strasberg in the Group Theatre and in the world-famous Actors Studio, all of which in a paradoxical manner carried the ideas of early Stanislavsky to a new level. It would be interesting to undertake a contemporary all-embracing examination of the basic element of the System – affective (emotional) memory – in order to understand to what degree various types of people are endowed with it, and to elaborate contemporary methods for its development. One would like to believe that the results of research into these various under-investigated issues will appear in the near future. All of this is necessary, among other things, in order that theatre practitioners and scholars understand the convention of dividing the System into early and late periods, and in order that they realize the organic unity of the Stanislavsky System.

---

[6] It was Robert Ellermann from whom I first heard the definition of the early period of the System as *basic*. I am glad for the opportunity here to thank him wholeheartedly for his generous support of my research on the development of the Stanislavsky System in the work of Lee Strasberg.

The present study is devoted to only one, but highly important, source for the System, a source that in many ways moulded its formation in the early period and fundamentally determined its subsequent development. This source is the teaching and practice of Yoga, an ancient Indian philosophy originating as far back as the third millennium BCE.

At the same time, the subject 'Stanislavsky and Yoga' itself is only part of a broader topic, namely the exploration of the influence of Yoga (both classical Yoga and modern yoga) and the Eastern psychophysical techniques on actor training of the twentieth century, a topic which deserves its own study. It should be carried out taking into account the creative achievements of many theoreticians and practitioners in world theatre, among which undoubtedly are the works of Jerzy Grotowski, Eugenio Barba, Peter Brook, and Richard Schechner. But it is precisely the creative practice of Konstantin Stanislavsky and his System that began the dialogue between East and West in the realm of theatrical culture and actor training.

It is also necessary to emphasize that understanding the interrelationship of actor training according to Stanislavsky and the centuries-old practice of Yoga will lead us beyond the problems of theatrical pedagogy. This understanding can illuminate fundamental problems of creativity in many spheres, as well as important questions of contemporary psychophysical practices for the self-improvement of man in general.

Translator's Note

In this text, I have anglicized Russian names (Stanislavsky, Tolstoy, Dostoevsky, Bely, Rimsky-Korsakov) according to guidelines established by the American Association of Teachers of Slavic and East European Languages and in keeping with the transliterations that are most familiar to English speakers. If in a quotation a name appears transliterated differently, then I retain that spelling. Otherwise, I follow the Library of Congress system of transliteration, with the following exceptions: established spellings of Russian scholars who have published in English (e.g. Anatoly Smeliansky, Sergei Tcherkasski) and of émigré Russians (e.g. Michael Chekhov, Maria Ouspenskaya, Andrius Jilinsky).

All authors' names in the footnotes with bibliographical information are written in the following form: 'Name Surname' – for English-language editions; and 'N[ame]. P[atronymic]. Surname' – for Russian-language editions. This indicates the origin of the books and how they are presented (and thus easily found) in the language of their publication.

Thus, for example, the name of Tcherkasski will appear in two forms: Sergei Tcherkasski for English-language editions and S. D. Tcherkasski for Russian-language editions.

Today the word 'Yoga' is written in two ways – 'Yoga' and 'yoga'. Some authors use 'Yoga' (Sharon Carnicke, Andrew White, Elizabeth De Michelis), some 'yoga' (Rose Whyman, Maria Kapsali). There is also the view that if one is referring to yoga as a specific Hindu philosophy, then it should be capitalized: 'Yoga'. But if it is just a matter of training (doing certain poses, stretches, etc.), then lower case is better: 'yoga'.

The author and translator of this book feel that it is important to distinguish between classical Yoga and yoga as a generic term. In view of the fact that in the books by Ramacharaka (the main source of yogic information for Stanislavsky) the first letter of the word is capitalized, in this book we will write mainly 'Yoga'. When we use 'yoga', the word refers to a contemporary system of exercises.

In producing this volume, the author referred directly to the original Russian texts and I translated all quotations from those original Russian texts specifically for this volume.

Introduction

In 1930, Stanislavsky wrote to his editor Liubov Gurevich about his nearly finished book *An Actor's Work on Himself*:[7]

> In my opinion, the main danger in this book is 'creation of the life of the human spirit' (one must not speak about the spirit). Other dangers: the subconscious, emanation, immanation, the word *soul*. Won't they prohibit the book because of that?[8]

Stanislavsky had reason to be afraid. In the late 1920s there began a forcible transformation of the Moscow Art Theatre into a model theatre, an element of the official picture of prosperity. Stalin's ideologues were creating 'a tower of socialist realism' out of the Art Theatre. A committee was formed to read Stanislavsky's book and to remove from the manuscript everything that did not meet the demands of materialistic philosophy, i.e. dialectical materialism.

They forced Stanislavsky into self-censorship. For instance, it was necessary to remove 'affective' memory. 'Now this term has been rejected and not replaced with a new one', says the author of the System in *An Actor's Work on Himself* and exclaims almost desperately, 'But we still need some word to define the concept [...].'[9] Thus 'affective' memory became 'emotional' memory. In his notebooks Stanislavsky even finds a 'translation' for his basic definition of the goal of dramatic art without using the word 'spirit' which was threatened by

[7]   Three major Stanislavsky books on actor training are known in the West under the titles that belong to the translator Elizabeth Hapgood, not to Stanislavsky himself. Stanislavsky's Russian-language title *An Actor's Work on Himself. Part I. An Actor's Work on Himself in the Creative Process of Experiencing* in the US edition of 1936 became *An Actor Prepares*; *An Actor's Work on Himself. Part II. An Actor's Work on Himself in the Creative Process of Embodiment* was published as *Building a Character* (1949), and *An Actor's Work on a Role* – as *Creating a Role* (1961). Out of these three books Stanislavsky authorized only the first one, the other two were compiled out of his drafts and numerous unfinished materials after his death. Translations by Jean Benedetti, *An Actor's Work* (2008) and *An Actor's Work on a Role* (2010), not only restore the original titles of Stanislavsky's books in English, but also fulfil his original plan of publishing the first two books in one volume.
[8]   Letter to L. Ia. Gurevich, 23 December 1930, in K. S. Stanislavskii, *Sobranie sochinenii* (Collected Works), 8 vols (Moscow: Iskusstvo, 1954–1961), VIII, 277–78, hereafter referred to as Stanislavskii, *Ss* 8.
[9]   Stanislavskii, *Ss* 9, II (1989), 279.

censorship: 'Instead of "creation of the life of the human spirit" [I could write] "creation of the inner world of the characters and conveying the idea of this world through artistic form".'[10] One can find an abundance of such compromises made by Stanislavsky in an attempt to deliver his most important thoughts and still get the approval of the censors.

At the same time an official from the Central Committee of the Communist Party, Alexei Angarov, politely but insistently 'instructed' the author of the System:

> Reading your published works and your manuscripts, leads me more and more to the conclusion that by 'intuition' you mean artistic instinct. One should explain vague terms, such as 'intuition' and 'subconscious', and show their realistic content. People should be told precisely what this artistic instinct is, and how it is expressed. This is one of the tasks of those who explore theoretically the questions of art.[11]

In that manner and without any hesitation, Angarov patronizingly explained the theory of art to the creator of the science of acting. Stanislavsky humbly thanked Angarov for the 'friendly' advice which he tried to follow (as indicated in his letter of 11 February 1937):

> In anticipation of our meeting where you will give me a detailed explanation about intuition, I cut out this word from the first edition [...] I agree that there is nothing mysterious or mystical about the creative process, and we should talk about that.[12]

In the late 1920s, all, or almost all, mention of philosophy and the practice of Yoga disappeared from Stanislavsky's manuscripts and published works. According to Stalin's ideologues, the great man of socialist realism in theatre

[10] K. S. Stanislavskii, *Iz zapisnykh knizhek*, 2 vols (Moscow: VTO, 1986), II, 323.

[11] Cited in V. V. Dybovskii, 'V plenu predlagaemykh obstoyatelstv', *Minuvshee: Istoricheskii almanakh*, X (1992), 312–13.

[12] Stanislavskii, *Ss* 8, VIII (1961), 432–33. To give a clearer picture of the tragic period of the 1930s it is worth mentioning that Alexei Angarov (1898–1937), Vice-Head of the Cultural Department of the Communist Party's Central Committee was executed in November of 1937.

could not derive inspiration from the mystical teaching of Indian hermits. Thus began the silencing of one of the most important sources of the System. The word 'Yoga' is already absent in *My Life in Art* (1926), and it is also not found in the Russian edition of *An Actor's Work on Himself in the Creative Process of Experiencing* (1938). It turns up fleetingly in the third volume of Stanislavsky's eight-volume *Collected Works* (1955), and only in the commentary explaining that 'the term "prana", borrowed from the philosophy of Hindu yogis, has been replaced with a clearer and more scientific term "muscular energy" or simply "energy".'[13]

The fourth volume of Stanislavsky's *Collected Works* (1957), *An Actor's Work on a Role*, gives more evidence of the connections between the Stanislavsky System and Yoga that evaded censorship. References to Yoga appear three times: in the statement that 'the only approach to the subconscious is through consciousness',[14] and in two vividly yogic examples: about the hidden work of the cluster of thoughts thrown into 'the bag of the subconscious' and about the silly child 'who, having planted a seed, pulls it out every half an hour in order to see whether it has put down roots'.[15] However, such few and scattered references sound more like individual fragments of Eastern fairy-tales, rather than a methodically grounded account of borrowings from the philosophy and practice of Yoga. As a result, the significance of the influence of the centuries-old yogic knowledge about the nature of man on the Stanislavsky System was constantly disparaged and even concealed in Soviet theatre studies, and usually rather aggressively. For example, in the book *The Stanislavsky System and Soviet Theatre* we read:

> In realistic theatre there is not and cannot be any place for Buddhism with its mystical, reactionary ravings. An enthusiasm for yogis is one of the obvious examples of how negatively

13 Stanislavskii, *Ss 8*, III (1955), 459.
14 Stanislavskii, *Ss 8*, IV (1957), 156.
15 *Ibid.*, 158–59.

the years of reaction affected the formation of the System. Stanislavsky had to free it from alien, idealistic influences.[16]

Valerii Galendeev justly concludes:

They liked to write about Stanislavsky, especially in the fifties and sixties, that at the turn of the century and during the first ('decadent') decade of the twentieth century, allegedly, he went through a brief and superficial infatuation with the philosophy of Indian yogis and their teaching about *prana* – a mysterious inner psychic substance that serves to make a connection between the human soul and the cosmos (or, if we translate this into the language more similar to that of the early Moscow Art Theatre, the World Soul).[17] They thought that Stanislavsky quickly and successfully got over the influence of the philosophy of distant Hindus and converted it all into the materialistic concept of action where there was no place for any 'mysticism'.[18]

In the present study I am trying to demonstrate the opposite.

In 1967, Sergei Gippius published his renowned collection of exercises, *The Gymnastics of Feelings*, based on Stanislavsky's practice. Although many of the exercises were taken directly from Yoga, which Gippius indicates in the introduction, the book does not contain any substantial analysis of Yoga's influence on the Stanislavsky System. The tone of the conversation about Yoga as a 'religious-idealistic philosophical system' is necessarily negative, at times even condescendingly ironic. The author ridicules the assumption about the presence of auras in man and reduces *prana* to a 'muscular feeling'.[19] For instance, Gippius, citing Pavel Simonov, mistakenly tries to reduce the phenomena of the 'emission of rays' and the

---

[16] N. A. Abalkin, *Sistema Stanislavskogo i sovetskii teatr,* 2nd edn (Moscow: Iskusstvo, 1954), 117.

[17] Galendeev refers here to the World Soul from Treplev's play in *The Seagull* by Anton Chekhov.

[18] V. N. Galendeev, *Uchenie Stanislavskogo o tsenicheskom slove* (Leningrad: LGITMiK, 1990), 105.

[19] S. V. Gippius, *Gimnastika chuvstv. Trening tvorcheskoi psikhotekhniki* (Leningrad and Moscow: Iskusstvo, 1967), 26.

'reception of rays'[20] to 'micromimic'.[21] In the second edition, prepared after the pedagogue's death in 1981, but published only in 2006, the more odious formulations are removed and a small chapter 'Yoga. T. Ribot. Traditions of Russian Realism' is allotted to a short account of Yoga. It starts with the confession that 'Yoga, the ancient Indian philosophical system, served as a stimulus to the creation of certain exercises',[22] and further the text contains a series of yogic tenets and exercises with an indication of their sources. However, even here the readers are told that, judging 'by Stanislavsky's last notes concerning training, his exercises of the 1930s were already free from [...] the mysticism of Yoga'.[23]

Thus even Gippius's latest book, largely relying on yogic training, does not contain a serious analysis of the connections between the Stanislavsky System and the teaching of Yoga. Moreover, unfortunately such an analysis still does not exist in Russian theatre studies today. The creators of websites about Yoga, proud of the famous people who practised Hatha Yoga, mention Stanislavsky, 'whose System, *as is well known, is based on Yoga* [italics are mine]'.[24] Who knows that? How is it based? Their claim, of course, is more an advertisement

[20] 'Emission of rays' and 'reception of rays' (*lucheispuskanie* and *luchevospriyatie*) – terms of the System introduced by Stanislavsky in the chapter 'Communication' of *An Actor's Work*. To convey the meaning of these terms translator Elizabeth Hapgood (*An Actor Prepares*, 1936) uses words 'rays' and 'irradiation' but generally avoids translating them, and cuts them out of her translation. Jean Benedetti (*An Actor's Work*, 2008) translates them as 'emitting and receiving rays'. The terms have also been translated as 'emanation' or 'radiation' and as 'irradiation' or 'immanation' (Carnicke, *Stanislavsky in Focus*, 1998, 2009).
[21] S. V. Gippius, *Gimnastika*, 282–83.
[22] S. V. Gippius, *Akterskii trening. Gimnastika chuvstv* (Saint Petersburg: Praim-Evroznak, 2006), 290.
[23] *Ibid.*, 292.
[24] On the website http://yogaclassic.ru/post/2128 in the work by A. P. Ocha-povskii 'Kriya-ioga i Xatxa-ioga dlia nachinaiushchikh', we read: 'Not only did Mahatma Gandhi and Jawaharlal Nehru engage in Hatha Yoga, but also the former US President John Kennedy, and in the Soviet Union, Konstantin Stanislavsky and others. The Nobel Prize laureate academician Ivan Pavlov also had a positive attitude towards yoga.'

than a reflection of the knowledge produced by modern theatre scholarship.

The absence of understanding of the interrelation between the Stanislavsky System and Yoga teaching leads to a series of problems in theatre pedagogy. Larisa Gracheva, an expert on actor 'training and drill',[25] justly points out that without the knowledge of the underlying yogic basis of individual exercises their goals become oversimplified, and their content vapid. Here is an example that she provides:

> The exercise 'listening to sounds' is almost always done in the first semester. However, its performance is often misunderstood: the 'unfortunate' students are told to listen to all the sounds in the room and outside of it, and the one who afterwards can list more sounds than his colleagues is supposedly more attentive. This exercise has ancient Zen roots, it was born from sound-based meditation and consisted not of remembering the greatest number of sounds, but in maximum concentration, of a change of consciousness where sounds fill one's consciousness, and one listens not only to the sounds, but also to *the spaces between them*. It is a very difficult exercise, requiring a certain degree of preparedness, and we offer it to newcomers who are in the first year of their studies. Naturally, the exercise quickly turns into a rather boring game; it is not absorbed and, above all, does not give results.[26]

---

[25] The notion of 'training and drill' was explained by Stanislavsky in the Preface for the Russian edition of *An Actor's Work* (1938). From the early 1910s he was planning to compile a workbook of practical exercises for actor training that would accompany each part of his books. Stanislavsky insisted that the System should enter into the student's classes and the actor's practice through a rigorous system of exercises designed to tune the actor's instrument. He called this training 'training and drill' (*trening i mushtra*) borrowing the term 'drill' (*mushtra*) from military vocabulary to underline the exacting nature of actor training. In order to indicate the two meanings of the English word 'training' – training as an educational process, and training as a system of exercises (*trening*) – 'training and drill' or *trening* will be used instead of 'training' where it is important to underline that it is a notion belonging to the System.

[26] L. V. Gracheva, 'Psikhotekhnika aktera v processe obucheniia: teoriia i praktika' (D.Sc. dissertation in Theatre Studies, Saint Petersburg State Theatre Arts Academy, 2005), 34–35.

This and many other examples demonstrate that today, a hundred years after Stanislavsky started to enrich the System with ideas drawn from Yoga, it is necessary to examine what the System really owes to ancient Indian philosophy and practice.

Although certain claims about the fundamental and long-term influence of Yoga on Stanislavsky started to penetrate Russian scholarship on theatre quite a while ago,[27] research of this subject was first done by non-Russian authors. Among substantial works we should name articles by William Wegner,[28] Andrew White,[29] and chapters from the books by Mel Gordon,[30] Sharon Carnicke,[31] and Rose Whyman.[32]

The present book arose as a result of my research carried out in 2007–08. Its first results were published in the Russian language journal *Voprosy teatra* (Questions of Theatre) in

---

[27] E. I. Poliakova, *Stanislavskii* (Moscow: Iskusstvo, 1977); E. I. Chernaia, *Kurs treninga fonatsionnogo dykhaniia i fonatsii na osnove uprazhnenii Vostoka* (Saint Petersburg: SPbGATI, 1997); I. I. Silanteva and Y. G. Klimenko, *Akter i ego Alter Ego* (Moscow: Graal, 2000). I would like to express my gratitude to Liubov Alferova for drawing my attention to the latter work and for reading and discussing the first version of my article that constitutes earlier material for this book.

[28] William H. Wegner, 'The Creative Circle: Stanislavski and Yoga', *Educational Theatre Journal*, 28 (1) (1976), 85–89.

[29] Andrew White, 'Stanislavsky and Ramacharaka: The Influence of Yoga and Turn-of-the-Century Occultism on the System', *Theater Survey*, 47 (1) (2006), 73–92. I consider it a pleasant duty to thank Andrew White for providing me with a copy of his article. A later version of this article appeared as the chapter 'Stanislavsky and Ramacharaka: The Impact of Yoga and the Occult Revival of the System' in *The Routledge Companion to Stanislavsky*, ed. by R. Andrew White (London and New York: Routledge, 2014), 287–304.

[30] Mel Gordon, *The Stanislavsky Technique: Russia* (New York: Applause Theatre Book Publishers, 1987), 30–37.

[31] Sharon Marie Carnicke, *Stanislavsky in Focus* (The Netherlands: Harwood Academic Publishers, 1998), 138–145; Sharon Marie Carnicke, *Stanislavsky in Focus: An Acting Master for the Twenty-First Century*, 2nd edn (London: Routledge, 2009), 167–84. I also had the opportunity to listen to the presentation by Sharon Carnicke at the symposium 'Stanislavsky in Finland' in April 2009 where both of us delivered papers. I am pleased to express my appreciation to her for the very interesting scholarly discussions that followed.

[32] Rose Whyman, *The Stanislavsky System of Acting: Legacy and Influence in Modern Performance* (Cambridge: Cambridge University Press, 2008), 78–88.

2009–2010,[33] and then appeared in the English language e-journal *Stanislavski Studies* in 2012–2013.[34] Further research resulted in my Russian language book *Stanislavsky and Yoga* published in 2013.[35]

Luckily, interest in the subject of Stanislavsky and his connections with Yoga and more generally the application of yoga in actor training continues to grow, and after my first publications, Elena Chernaia, who was teaching voice and speech at my Acting Studio in the Saint Petersburg Theatre Arts Academy produced a textbook devoted to the use of the breathing gymnastics of Yoga in the education of actors,[36] and Maria Kapsali defended her dissertation entitled 'The Use of Yoga in Actor Training and Theatre Making'.[37] My own interest in the topic also keeps growing, and I have enjoyed finding some more materials for this English edition of the book as well as doing practical workshops and presentations about Stanislavsky and Yoga in recent times.

Naturally, I have used some of the ideas from the earlier research by Carnicke, White, and Whyman during work on this book. However, the main source is, of course, the literary legacy and practice of Stanislavsky himself.

[33]   S. D. Tcherkasski, 'Stanislavskii i ioga: opyt parallelnogo chteniia', *Voprosy teatra; Proscaenium*, 3–4 (2009), 282–300. S. D. Tcherkasski, 'Iogicheskie element sistemy Stanislavskogo', *Voprosy teatra; Proscaenium*, 1–2 (2010), 252–70.

[34]   Sergei Tcherkasski, 'Fundamentals of the Stanislavski System and Yoga Philosophy and Practice', *Stanislavski Studies*, 1 (2012), 1–18 <http://stanislavskistudies.org/category/issues/issue-1/>; Sergei Tcherkasski, 'Fundamentals of the Stanislavski System and Yoga Philosophy and Practice, Part 2', *Stanislavski Studies*, 2 (2013), 190–236 <http://stanislavskistudies.org>.

[35]   S. D. Tcherkasski, *Stanislavskii i ioga* (Saint Petersburg: SPbGATI, 2013).

[36]   E. I. Chernaia, *Vospitanie fonatsionnogo dykhaniia s ispolzovaniem printsipov dykhatelnoi gimnastiki 'iogi'* (Moscow: Granitsa, 2009).

[37]   Maria Kapsali, 'The Use of Yoga in Actor Training and Theatre Making' (unpublished Ph.D. dissertation in Performance Practice [Drama], University of Exeter, 2010), 294. See also Maria Kapsali, 'The Presence of Yoga in Stanislavski's Work,' *Stanislavski Studies*, 3 (2013), 139–50 <http://stanislavskistudies.org>. I am very grateful to Maria Kapsali for providing me with copies of her other articles (see Bibliography).

CHAPTER I

Yoga in the Theatre Practice
of Stanislavsky

Stanislavsky's Acquaintance
with Yoga

Stanislavsky was introduced to the teaching of yogis in 1911. This moment is recorded in detail in the memoirs of actress Nadezhda Smirnova about her vacations together with Stanislavsky's family in Saint-Lunaire, France, in the summer of 1911. She recollects that Nikolai Demidov,[38] the tutor of Stanislavsky's son, was often present during the everyday conversations 'by the deep blue sea', during which Stanislavsky tested his thoughts about the System on his listeners. This medical student from Moscow University, who also studied Tibetan medicine at the Saint Petersburg Russian-Buryat school of Piotr Badmaiev, doctor to the Tsar's family,[39] upon listening to Stanislavsky once told him:

> 'Why should you yourself invent exercises and search for the names of things that have been named long, long ago. I will give you books. Read *Hatha Yoga* and *Raja Yoga*. That will interest you, because many of your thoughts coincide with the things written there.' Indeed, Stanislavsky became interested, and it seems that these books confirmed and clarified many of his own discoveries in the sphere of the psychology of creative work on stage.[40]

[38] Nikolai Demidov (1884–1953) – theatrical teacher, director, assistant, but subsequently opponent of Stanislavsky. His first book was published after his death in 1965; and only at the beginning of the twenty-first century his four-volume collection of works on actor training was published.

[39] T. I. Grekova, 'Tibetskaia meditsina v Rossii', *Nauka i religiia*, 8 (1988), 11.

[40] Cited in *Zhizn i tvorchestvo K. S. Stanislavskogo: Letopis v chetyrekh tomax*, ed. by I. N. Vinogradskaia, 4 vols (Moscow: Moskovskii khudozhestvennyi teatr, 2003), II, 291–92. The memoirs of Vadim Shverubovich also contain an indirect story about this episode. The son of Vasilii Kachalov writes about the tutor of the sixteen-year-old Igor Alekseev, whom the children nicknamed 'Tsyfirkin' (Tsyfirkin, a character in the famous Russian play *The Minor* by Fonvizin, a retired soldier who has become a teacher, is a negative name for a strict teacher). This teacher of Stanislavsky's son was 'an alumnus of the medical department [of Moscow University], a young athletic doctor, wrestler and judge of French (classical) wrestling, Nikolai Vasilevich Demidov'. He 'was enthusiastic about yogis and their school of the physical and spiritual education of man' and he tormented his pupil with demands for correct and slow chewing of food in accordance with the yogic doctrine of health. See V. V. Shverubovich, *O liudiakh, o teatre i o sebe* (Moscow: Iskusstvo, 1976), 97–98.

Smirnova is right in her conclusions. Having returned to Moscow, Stanislavsky indeed acquired a Russian version of Ramacharaka's book, *Hatha Yoga: Yogic Philosophy of the Physical Well-Being of Man*, translated and edited by V. Singh (Saint Petersburg, 1909), and thoroughly studied it, as is evidenced by the copy with his notes that is in the Museum of the Moscow Art Theatre.[41]

However, according to some sources, Stanislavsky might have become acquainted with the ideas of Indian philosophers earlier. This is not surprising: an interest in the East permeated Russian art of the turn of the century. Lev Tolstoy, whose influence on Stanislavsky was considerable, for many years corresponded with Gandhi.[42] The reading of many individuals – the philosopher Vladimir Solovyev, the poet Maximilian Voloshin, the composer Alexander Skriabin, the writer Andrei Bely – included classics of the East: *Mahabharata*, *The Upanishads*, *The Vedas*. After the war with Japan and the relaxation of censorship following the revolution of 1905, interest in the East led to the development of schools of occult philosophy, which to a large degree relied on Hindu religion in general, and on Yoga in particular. The mystical teaching of Georgii Gurdjieff (1866?–1949), freely deriving its elements from Islam, Yoga, and even numerology, or the theosophy dependent on Brahmanism and Buddhism as interpreted by, among others, Elena Blavatskaia (Helena

[41] Ramacharaka, *Khatkha-ioga*, Archive of the Museum of the Moscow Art Theatre, K. S. Stanislavsky Collection, no. 11262.

[42] For example, in Lev Tolstoy's diary for July 31, 1896, there is a note: 'during this time there was a letter from the Hindu Tod and a charming book of Hindu wisdom *Joga's Philosophy*'. See L. N. Tolstoy, *Polnoe sobranie sochinenii*, 90 vols (Moscow: Goslitizdat [Gosudarstvennoe izdatel'stvo khudozhestvennoi literatury]: 1955), LIII, 106. The book mentioned was *Joga's Philosophy: Lectures on Raja Joga or Conquering Internal Nature* by Swami Vivekananda (New York: Advaita Ashrama, 1896), which was published in 1911 in the Russian translation of Ia. K. Popov already after Tolstoy's death under the title *Filosofiia ioga. Lektsii, chitannye v Niu-Iorke zimoiu 1895-1896; o Radzhi-ioge, ili podchinenii vnutrennei prirody, aforizmy Patandzhali s kommentariiami*. See also A. I. Shifman, *Lev Tolstoi i Vostok* (Moscow: Nauka, 1971).

Blavatsky) (1831–1891), can serve as examples. The Russian Theosophy Society was organized in 1908, and Nikolai Roerich (1874–1947), who was one of its members, was well known to Stanislavsky since he designed sets and costumes for *Peer Gynt* at the Moscow Art Theatre in 1912. Subsequently, Roerich and his wife, Elena Roerich (1879–1955), spending years travelling around Tibet and India, created their own interpretation of yogic philosophy which acquired the name of the Hindu god of fire, Agni-Yoga. Maxim Gorky, a constant interlocutor of Stanislavsky during the early period of the maturing of the System, became acquainted with the works of Blavatskaia by 1899 and, although at first sceptical about the ideas of theosophy, in 1912 fought for the publication of all of her works in Russian.[43]

One could multiply the examples: many Russian artists of this period, disillusioned by the spiritual apathy of society, turned to the ideas of the East, seeing in them a counterweight to the growing industrialization and the standardizing materialism of Western consciousness. According to the data of the journal of the ecumenical movement, by 1913 in Russia there were thirty five active occult organizations, and in the period from 1881 to 1918 there arose nearly thirty esoteric journals.[44]

The history of the Order of the Templars (Order of the Light), among whose knights were many of the creative people of Moscow in the 1920s and 1930s, including actors and directors of the Moscow Art Theatre and its studios (e.g. Yury Zavadsky, Ruben Simonov, Valentin Smyshliaev, Alexander

[43]   Information for this paragraph is derived from White, 76–77, where works of Russian scholars that appeared in English are cited: Roman Lunkin and Sergei Filatov, 'The Rerikh Movement: A Homegrown Russian "New Religious Movement"', *Religion, State & Society*, 28 (1) (2000), 135–48; Oleg Maslenikov, *The Frenzied Poets: Andrey Biely and the Russian Symbolists* (Berkeley and Los Angeles: University of California Press, 1952), 128–31. See also Bernice Glatzer Rosenthal, 'Introduction' in *The Occult in Russian and Soviet Culture*, ed. by B. G. Rosenthal (Ithaca: Cornell University Press, 1997), 21–23.
[44]   John McCannon, 'In Search of Primeval Russia: Stylistic Evolution in the Landscapes of Nicholas Roerich, 1897–1914', *Cultural Geographies*, 7 (3) July (2000), 272.

Blagonravov, Lidiia Deikyn, and others) might illustrate how serious the interest in Eastern philosophy was in Russia even in the post-revolutionary period. It gives a vivid picture of how firm these enthusiasms were as well as what unusual combinations of Western and Eastern esoteric thought arose in the spiritual practice of Russian theatre people.[45]

As is evident from the above, Yoga penetrated into the consciousness of the intelligentsia, not in its own right, but very often combined with other philosophical and religious views. Each thinker took what he needed from the centuries-old Indian practice, and Stanislavsky himself behaved exactly the same, grafting the experience of Yoga onto his System.

According to A. L. Fovitzky, yogic techniques attracted Stanislavsky's attention already in 1906, when he found himself unable to concentrate on the thoughts of the character while he performed the role of Astrov in *Uncle Vanya* (Stanislavsky himself, describing a similar episode, mentions Ibsen's *Doctor Stockmann*).[46] It was precisely then that Stanislavsky

> found a hint in the practice of the Buddhist wise men – and thenceforth he required his actors to practice prolonged psychophysical exercises as a means of cultivating concentration. Following the teachings of Eastern metaphysics, his followers strove to visualize the elusive 'I' – in order, while on the stage, to live the life of the spirit and to become acquainted with unknown sides of the spiritual life.[47]

Recalling in *My Life in Art* the rehearsals in 1908 for *A Month in the Country*, Stanislavsky used entirely yogic terminology as he wrote about his search for a method of revealing the 'soul of the actor' to the audience. He affirmed that 'some sort of invisible emanations of the creative will and

[45] S. D. Tcherkasski, *Valentin Smyshliaev – akter, rezhisser, pedagog* (Saint Petersburg: SPbGATI, 2004), 26–30.
[46] Stanislavskii, *Ss* 9, I (1988), 371–72.
[47] A. L. Fovitzky, *The Moscow Art Theatre and Its Distinguishing Characteristics* (New York: Chernoff Publishing Co., 1923), 42.

feeling are necessary'.[48] However, a chronological inversion is possible here, for Stanislavsky in 1923 involuntarily described the essence of his searches of 1908 with the knowledge gained from a serious study of Yoga that followed later.

Probably, Leopold Sulerzhitsky also played a role in Stanislavsky's introduction to the philosophy of Hinduism. Sulerzhitsky was knowledgeable about Eastern spiritualism, and also, among numerous things he knew, about the practice of the Dukhobors[49]. It was after reading Sulerzhitsky's notes about the two-year saga of the transportation of the members of this religious sect to Canada that Stanislavsky invited 'Suler' to be his assistant.[50] The meditative practice of the Dukhobors that resonated with Eastern practice undoubtedly influenced the Tolstoyan Sulerzhitsky.

Some claim that Sulerzhitsky introduced Stanislavsky to morning meditation about upcoming projects of the day, which was a part of Dukhobor practice: they would sit in a relaxed position and mentally, step by step, imagine and visualize how they would fulfil each task of the day that lay ahead.[51] Of course, that does not prove the acquaintance of Stanislavsky with this practice, but it is worth pointing out Stanislavsky's similar descriptions of an actor's mental journey in the process of 'perceiving the role'. In *An Actor's Work on a Role* (*Woe from Wit*), an actor imagines the circumstances and tasks of his role and, 'dreaming about the role', enters Famusov's house, meets people there, and even establishes contact with them.[52]

But, if the evidence of Stanislavsky's early interest in Yoga is fragmentary and in part conjectures, the fact that Stanislavsky

[48]   Stanislavskii, *Ss* 9, I (1988), 406.
[49]   The Dukhobors (literally 'Spirit Wrestlers') are a Spiritual Christian religious group that originated in Russia in the eighteenth century. Their rejection of the Orthodox Church and government interference in their life led to an exodus of the majority of the Dukhobors from Russia in 1898–99.
[50]   Suler was a nickname of Leopold Sulerzhitsky which was used by nearly everybody in the Moscow Art Theatre.
[51]   Gordon, 31–32.
[52]   Stanislavskii, *Ss* 9, IV (1991), 72–85.

started to use Yoga after 1911 – the year he became acquainted with Ramacharaka's *Hatha Yoga* – is beyond doubt. The site for the inculcation of ancient Indian practice to actor training of the twentieth century was the First Studio of the Art Theatre.

Yoga in the First Studio of the Moscow Art Theatre

The record of one of Stanislavsky's lessons conducted in the First Studio in late autumn of 1913 gives an idea of the nature of the utilization of yogic principles in the training of young actors.[53] Stanislavsky had started by conducting a series of experiments with the students: 'I compelled everyone to do "the last day of Pompeii".[54] They began to yell. Everyone's muscles became tense', wrote Stanislavsky and further on: 'I argued that it is not possible to make even simple calculations with tension in the muscles. Everyone was tense, nobody could mentally perform simple arithmetic.'[55] So Stanislavsky suggested the Yoga experience as a solution to the problem of excess muscular tension. Therefore, a separate point in the lesson was: 'About Hatha Yoga (cat, rest, nirvana)'.[56] Then Stanislavsky engaged in practical exercises against excess tension of the muscles ('Not relaxation, but release', he warned against the typical mistakes of students).[57] He introduced the concepts of an inner observer, of the object of attention, and of the circle of attention. ('The diaphragm of a photographer: a big one, the size of the whole auditorium, and a small one, a small circle [...]. A visual circle; an aural circle; a sensual circle.'[58])

[53]   The First Studio was founded in September 1912, performed its first show in January 1913 and officially opened to the public in November 1913. In 1924 it became the Second Moscow Art Theatre; it was closed in 1936.
[54]   Improvisation based on the famous epic painting 'The Last Day of Pompeii' by Russian artist Karl Briullov (1799–1852).
[55]   Stanislavskii, *Ss* 9, V, Book 2 (1994), 376.
[56]   *Ibid.*
[57]   *Ibid.*, 377.
[58]   *Ibid.*

Although not many of this kind of record of Stanislavsky's lessons have been preserved, one should not doubt the regularity of yogic classes. As Elena Poliakova, reconstructing a working day of the Studio members, wrote: 'improvisations alternated with readings from *Hatha Yoga*'.[59]

In the First Studio, this book was passed around and became required reading. A letter by Evgeny Vakhtangov to his colleagues in May 1915 states:

> There is one more request. Take 1 ruble from the cash register on my account. Buy Ramacharaka's *Hatha Yoga*. And give it to Ekzempliarskaia on my behalf [Vera Ekzempliarskaia was a student in the First Studio]. She should read the book attentively and in the summer she must do the exercises from the part on breathing and on 'prana'.[60]

Vakhtangov also requested a report from Ekzempliarskaia herself: 'When you have read *Hatha Yoga*, write to me. Please.'[61] Of course the unusual Yoga books gave a new view on the surrounding world, on the lore of acting, and could not help but arouse the curiosity of young actors. 'We were never silent except on the stage or in classes', recalled later the actor and director of the First Studio Richard Boleslavsky and he shared the main themes of the Studio's discussions in this way: 'We disputed hotly about the origin of Rhythm, or the Coordination between the Mind and the Emotions, or Yogi culture applied to the Art of Acting.'[62]

The memoirs of another participant of the Studio, Boris Sushkevich,[63] about one of the rehearsals in 1912 (in this case

---

[59] E. I. Poliakova, *Teatr Sulerzhitskogo: Etika. Estetika. Rezhissura* (Moscow: Agraf, 2006), 184.

[60] Evgenii Vakhtangov, *Sbornik* (Moscow: VTO, 1984), 211. *Evgenii Vakhtangov. Dokumenty i svidetelstva*, 2 vols, ed. by V. V. Ivanov (Moscow: Indrik, 2011), II, 93. It is noteworthy that in the Vakhtangov library itself, the following Yoga books are preserved: Iog Ramacharaka, *Zhnani-Ioga* (Saint Petersburg, 1914); Iog Ramacharaka, *Puti dostizheniia indiiskikh iogov* (Saint Petersburg, 1915); Svami Vivekananda, *Karma-Ioga* (Saint Petersburg: Leontiev, 1914). See *Vakhtangov. Dokumenty*, II, 95.

[61] *Ibid.*, 212.

[62] Richard Boleslavsky, *Lances Down* (New York: Garden City, 1932), 55–56.

[63] Boris Sushkevich (1887–1946) – actor and director in the Moscow Art

he is talking about Anton Chekhov's short story 'The Witch') give us a picture of how the ideas, found in the Yoga books, were realized in practice:

> In the Studio on Tverskaia, in a very small room six to seven booths – in the literal sense of this word, like on the beach – are built. In each booth sits a couple: a sexton and a 'witch' [two main characters of the story]. They all rehearse simultaneously and do not disturb one another. To speak loudly is not allowed. When sound bursts out, it is incorrect. They only look at one another and whisper something […] it was forbidden to make a sound.[64]

Sushkevich was not able to say this openly (his memoir was published in 1933), but what he described is nothing other than a yogic exercise on the *emanation of prana*.

Freer in her expressions was another actress of the First Studio, Vera Soloviova.[65] Already in the United States, she recalled:

> We worked a great deal on concentration. It was called 'To go into the circle'. We imagined a circle around us and sent 'prana' rays of communication into the space and to each other for communication. Stanislavsky said 'send the prana here – I want to transmit it with the tips of my fingers. Send it to God, to the sky, or, afterwards, to your partner. I believe in my inner energy and I emit it – I spread it.'[66]

Michael Chekhov, who later became a follower of Rudolf Steiner's theosophy, claimed that in the 1910s he 'grasped the

Theatre and the First Studio; director of the famous production of the First Studio *Cricket on the Hearth* (1914); in the 1930s and 1940s artistic director of the Leningrad Academic Pushkin (Alexandrinskii) and Leningrad New (Novyi) Theatres, rector of the Leningrad Theatre Institute (now Saint Petersburg Theatre Arts Academy).

[64] B. M. Sushkevich, *Sem' momentov raboty nad roliu* (Leningrad: Gosudarstvennyi akademicheskii teatr dramy, 1933), 11.

[65] Vera Soloviova (1892–1986) – one of the leading actresses of the First Studio and the Second Moscow Art Theatre; in 1930 she left, together with her husband Andrius Jilinsky, first to Lithuania (they worked there with Michael Chekhov again), and then in 1935 to America, where she managed the Vera Soloviova Studio of Acting.

[66] Paul Gray, 'The Reality of Doing: Interviews with Vera Soloviova, Stella Adler, and Sanford Meisner', *Stanislavski and America*, ed. by Erika Munk (New York: Hill and Wang, 1966), 202.

philosophy of yogis quite openly, […] without the least inner resistance.'[67] For example, Chekhov regarded *emanation* as one of the most important devices of an actor's psycho-technique. Here is just one excerpt from his exercises. It is taken from *On the Technique of Acting* and coincides almost verbatim with Soloviova's memoirs about Stanislavsky's 'training and drill' (*trening*) in the First Studio: 'Start emanating your energy from your chest, then from your stretched out hands, and, finally, from your whole being. Send emanations in different directions.'[68] Chekhov paid a lot of attention to such work with *prana emanation*, and Beatrice Straight, his devoted student at Dartington Hall in England and during the American period, described Chekhov's exercises on radiation as 'beaming an aura… in an almost mystical sense'.[69]

Exploring the holistic triad 'consciousness, body, soul' in the creative sense of self of an actor, the training in the First Studio was largely given over to spiritual aspects. Primacy of the spiritual guidance over the purely technical *trening* was connected, in the first place, with the personality of Sulerzhitsky. With good reason did the participant of the Studio, Alexei Dikii,[70] note that Sulerzhitsky 'was not a director in the usual sense of the word' and that 'his influence on the production was realized through spiritual "prompting"'.[71] Also Stanislavsky recalled that his assistant dreamed that together they would 'create some kind of a spiritual order of actors'.[72]

---

[67] M. A. Chekhov, *Literaturnoe nasledie*, 2 vols (Moscow: Iskusstvo, 1986), I, 107.

[68] *Ibid.*, 260.

[69] Cited in Foster Hirsch, *A Method to Their Madness: The History of the Actors Studio*, 2nd edn (Cambridge MA: Da Capo, 2002), 347.

[70] Alexei Dikii (1889–1955) – actor and director in the First Studio and the Second Moscow Art Theatre, which he abandoned as a result of conflict with Michael Chekhov. Dikii directed in many theatres in Moscow and Leningrad, was repressed, and when he returned from the Gulag he played the role of Stalin on stage and in film; in the course of four years he received five Stalin prizes.

[71] A. D. Dikii, *Povest o teatralnoi iunosti* (Moscow: Iskusstvo, 1957), 214.

[72] Stanislavskii, *Ss* 9, I (1988), 437.

When the time came for the former actors and directors of the First Studio themselves to start teaching, they remembered the lessons of Suler. For instance, Richard Boleslavsky,[73] who, together with another participant of the First Studio, Maria Ouspenskaya,[74] founded the American Laboratory Theatre (The Lab), in his pedagogy also 'singled out the actor's spiritual training as the most important part of the work, and developed a series of what he called "soul exercises"'.[75] Ouspenskaya herself continued doing Yoga for her whole life and became a participant of the American society, the Self-Realization Fellowship, founded in 1920 by Paramahansa Yogananda, author of the book *Autobiography of a Yogi*.[76] It was Yogananda who led the funeral ceremony at the burial of Ouspenskaya on 6 December 1949.[77] According to White, in an informal talk to the Hollywood SRF congregation shortly after Ouspenskaya's death the famous yogi uttered a prayer for her soul, calling the actress and teacher 'one of our devoted followers' and a 'beloved student'.[78] (We also find reference to this side of her life in a book of a friend from her youth,

---

[73] Richard Boleslavsky (1889–1937) – actor and director in the Moscow Art Theatre and the First Studio; director of the first show of the First Studio, *The Good Hope*; key figure in the spreading of the Stanislavsky System in America; founder and artistic director of the Laboratory Theatre in New York; Hollywood director; author of the books *Acting: The First Six Lessons*, *Way of the Lancer* and *Lances Down*.

[74] Maria Ouspenskaya (1887–1949) – a former character actress of the Moscow Art Theatre and the First Studio, who conducted daily acting classes in the American Laboratory Theatre. In the 1930s and 1940s she continued her teaching in her own Maria Ouspenskaya Studio. She appeared on Broadway and in many films and twice was nominated for an Oscar.

[75] Hirsch, 63–64.

[76] Paramahansa Yogananda (1893–1952) was the most distinguished representative of kriya-yoga whose efforts helped to introduce many people in the Western World to yoga. After 1920 he lived in America, where in that same year he founded the Self-Realization Fellowship; in his book *Autobiography of a Yogi* (1946) he describes the ideal life of a yogi, dedicated to serving humanity. See White, 76, 80.

[77] Harlow Robinson, *Russians in Hollywood, Hollywood's Russians: Biography of an Image* (Boston: Northeastern University Press, 2007), 89.

[78] Paramahansa Yogananda, *One Life Versus Reincarnation*. Cited in White, 80.

Sofia Giatsintova;[79] stories reached Moscow that at the time of Ouspenskaya's funeral, 'Hindus in funeral clothes filled the street – as it turns out she belonged to their faith, and she was consecrated....'[80]) Although the degree of practical utilization of Yoga in the lessons of Ouspenskaya's acting class is not reliably known,[81] it is worth mentioning that Lee Strasberg, being a student in her classes at the American Laboratory Theatre, was making notes on Yoga fundamentals. His diary of 1924–1925 contains a full page of terms like *bhāva*, *vibhāva*, *sattvabhāva*, *sûnyatā*, as well as analysis of the structure of the Buddhist 'sevenfold office'.[82] Mel Gordon also writes about a special atmosphere in Ouspenskaya's lessons in the thirties: 'Madame [so Ouspenskaya was called by her American students] instilled a quietism and religiosity indoors. [...] Ouspenskaya began a class as if the group were young priests or nuns in a Buddhist monastery.'[83]

Another participant in the Studio, Valentin Smyshliaev,[84] a friend of Michael Chekhov, director of *Hamlet* in the Second Moscow Art Theatre, and Knight of the Templar Order of Light, also preserved an interest in Eastern esoterics throughout his whole creative life. I devoted the book *Valentin Smyshliaev – Actor, Director, Teacher* to an analysis of his teaching and directing and to the story of his unusual fate. The subtitle of the book is *The Teacher of*

---

[79]   Sofia Giatsintova (1895–1982) – leading actress of the First Studio and the Second Moscow Art Theatre, author of one of the most informative memoirs about the life of these theatres, *Alone With My Memory* (*S pamiatiu naedine*, 1985).
[80]   S. V. Giatsintova, *S pamiatiu naedine*, 2nd edn (Moscow: Iskusstvo, 1989), 177.
[81]   White, 76.
[82]   Lee Strasberg, *Notes from the Laboratory Theatre* in the file 'Lab Theatre', Archive of the Lee Strasberg Theatre and Film Institute (New York, 1924).
[83]   Mel Gordon, *Stanislavsky in America: An Actor's Workbook* (London: Routledge, 2010), 82.
[84]   Valentin Smyshliaev (1891–1936) – actor, director, theoretician of theatre. His book *Teoriia obrabotki stsenicheskogo zrelishcha* (1921) was one of the first attempts to set forth the Stanislavsky System, though the System's creator himself was sharply against this.

My Teacher, because my own teacher, Mar Vladimirovich
Sulimov, Professor of Directing at LGITMIK (the Leningrad
State Institute of Theatre, Music, and Cinematography, now
the Saint Petersburg State Theatre Arts Academy), studied in
Smyshliaev's Directing Studio at GITIS (the State Institute
of Theatre Art).[85] Thus I know first hand that the experience
of being introduced to Yoga in the First Studio remained with
many of its members for their whole life and was inevitably
passed along to the next generation of students.

Yoga in Stanislavsky's Classes with Actors
of the Moscow Art Theatre and the Second Studio
in the late 1910s and the 1920s

Having entered into the pedagogy of Stanislavsky and Sulerzhitsky in the First Studio, Yoga was successfully applied
by Stanislavsky later – in the subsequent training of students
in the Second Studio (created in 1916) and the Opera Studio
(created in 1918), as well as with the actors of the Moscow
Art Theatre itself. Stanislavsky's notebooks from the season
1919–1920 contain a considerable amount of notes about the
use of Hatha Yoga in the classes. It was practised together
with Swedish gymnastics, exercises on rhythm, Duncan's
gymnastics, speech training, and muscle relaxation. Diversity of exercises on an actor's external technique was balanced
with Stanislavsky's strict demand: '*Nota bene* once and for
all. Every single exercise should be motivated in advance or
justified by an inner psychological action or task.'[86]

In 'The Plan of Further Operatic Exercises' (October 1920)
we find the following instructions on muscle relaxation: 'Create
(in oneself) an unconscious observer of freedom. At first sitting,
lying (Hatha Yoga), then standing.'[87] Further, after a few pages:

[85]   See Tcherkasski, *Smyshliaev* (2004).
[86]   Stanislavskii, *Iz zapisnykh knizhek*, II (1986), 209.
[87]   *Ibid.*, 209–10.

During muscle relaxation there are two moments: a) release (recall) of prana and b) sending it. Prana (in Hindu – 'heart') releases (is being released) in order to act, to make use of this energy. Use it how and for what? First, in order to support the body's centre of gravity in all sorts of positions; second, in order to act not only with the body, muscles, eyes, ears, all the five senses, but with the soul as well.[88]

However, the most detailed connection with Yoga can be traced in the notes for the classes with actors of the Moscow Art Theatre. Analyzing Stanislavsky's lesson plan for the Moscow Art Theatre actors on 13 October 1919, Rose Whyman has paid attention to the fact that it contains a hidden synopsis of *Hatha Yoga*.[89] In giving an extensive quotation, following the British scholar, I will italicize and mark with square brackets the parallels between Stanislavsky's text and chapters of Ramacharaka's book, which was the main source of knowledge for the author of the System about the theory and practice of Yoga.

Stanislavsky wrote:

> We will be dealing with the art of experiencing [...]. The elements of this creative state: a) freedom of the body (the muscles), b) concentration, c) activeness.
>
> I am starting with muscle relaxation. Teaching about prana. a) Prana – the energy of life, is taken from the air [*Chapter XX. Pranic Energy*], food [*Chapter X. Prana Absorption from Food*], the sun [*Chapter XVII. The Solar Energy*], water [*Chapter XII. Irrigation of the Body*], human emanations. b) When a person dies, prana goes into the earth through worms, into microorganisms [*Chapter XVIII. The Little Lives of the Body*]. c) I, I am – not prana. This is that which unites all the pranas into one. d) How prana passes into the blood and nerves through the teeth, the chewing of food. How to breathe, to perceive unboiled water, sun rays. How to chew and breathe in order to receive more prana (to chew food so well that you drink it, not swallow it). [*Chapter X. Prana Absorption from Food*]. Breathe; six heartbeats – breathe in; three heartbeats – hold the air; and

[88] *Ibid.*, 213–14.
[89] Whyman, 83.

six heartbeats – breathe out. To reach up to fifteen heartbeats [...] [*Chapter XXI*. Pranic Exercises].

Sitting exercises. a) Sit and name the place which is tensed. b) Completely relax so that you can freely move your neck, etc. c) Do not stiffen into immobility. Listen to the movement of prana. d) The prana moves, shimmers like mercury, like a snake, from the hands to the fingertips, from the hip to the toes. e) The role of toes in walking. Throwing out the hips; the role of the spinal column. Exercise: swinging of a leg free as a whip from the hip and simultaneous raising and lowering on the toes. Same with the hands, same with the spinal column. f) Prana's movement is created, in my opinion, through inner rhythm [*Chapter XXI*. Pranic Exercises].[90]

The coincidences between the texts are indisputable, and in some places match exactly, including even the numbers used in counting (six – three – six – fifteen) suggested for breathing in, breathing out, and holding one's breath.

Thus, although Stanislavsky does not speak directly about *pranayama* (i.e. the division of Yoga that teaches the techniques for controlling *prana*), his notes reveal a serious study of the concepts of yogic practice. He boldly uses *pranayama* exercises in order to promote an actor's creative sense of self and genuine communication.

Moreover, Stanislavsky's fascination with Yoga only increased in the first post-revolutionary years, in the period when his research interests turned to the *external* technique of an actor and to the exploration of deep connections between the psyche and the physics of the actor in the process of creating.

The path of knowledge travelled by Michael Chekhov confirms the prevalence of the ideas of Yoga among Stanislavsky's students at the turn of the 1920s. He recalled:

I was carried away by yogis in my youth, beginning approximately at the age of 20 [i.e. 1911]. Vakhtangov and I studied them

---

[90] Stanislavskii, *Iz zapisnykh knizhek*, II (1986), 220–21.

together (although the word 'studied' is perhaps too serious and responsible [...]. Evgeny Bagrationovich [Vakhtangov] and I were *interested*, yogis disturbed us deeply).[91]

The actor wrote that 'for years I lived with the ideas of yogis, I got used to their worldview',[92] and he called the understanding of Hindu philosophy an 'illumination'. This understanding occurred only through the process of working with the students in his own so-called Chekhov Studio at the start of the 1920s.[93] Chekhov stated:

> I succeeded in understanding that the *creation of life* is the basic note of yogism. The creation of life! Here was that new note which gradually penetrated my soul. I began to look carefully at my past and look closely at the present. Perhaps there was no *creation of life* in the process of creating and conducting the Chekhov Studio? Perhaps the Studio of the Moscow Art Theatre was not created by K. S. Stanislavsky, L. A. Sulerzhitsky, and by us ourselves? Why, up to the present day, did I understand the term 'creative work' to mean only that which was done on stage? *The area of creativity began to expand for me* [italics are mine].[94]

Strictly speaking, behind this discovery of the 'truth known long ago' about the possibility of 'creativity within one's very self' is concealed the mature philosophical acceptance of the Stanislavsky System by Chekhov (as Stanislavsky often repeated, 'in our lore, to understand means to feel'[95]!) and the beginning of his own pedagogy. Only just having gotten to know 'the difference between a person creating *outside himself* and a person creating *within himself*',[96] the great actor

[91] Michael Chekhov, 'Letter to A. G. Bergstrem, Oct. 6, 1954' in M. A. Chekhov, *Literaturnoe nasledie*, 2 vols, 2nd edn (Moscow: Iskusstvo, 1995), I, 525.
[92] *Ibid.*, 526.
[93] In the 1920–21 season, Stanislavsky was conducting classes in four studios at once: Vakhtangov's, the Armenian Studio, the Habimah, and Chekhov's. Thus Chekhov had a chance not only to be trained by Stanislavsky as an actor but partially as an acting teacher as well.
[94] M. A. Chekhov, *Put Aktera* (The Path of the Actor) in M. A. Chekhov, *Literaturnoe nasledie* (1995), I, 89.
[95] Stanislavskii, *Ss* 9, I (1988), 373.
[96] M. A. Chekhov, *Put Aktera*, I, 89.

came out of a crisis which nearly led him to suicide. In the book, *The Path of the Actor*, he writes:

> I could not then understand this difference with the clarity with which it appears before me now. From experience, I knew about only one type of creation: outside oneself. It seemed to me that creative work is not subject to the will of man, and its direction depends exclusively on that so-called natural predisposition. But, together with the thought of *self-creation,* there naturally arose in me a volitional impulse – like a certain volitional rush towards mastery of creative energy – with the aim of transferring it inside, into myself.[97]

This was published in 1928, when Chekhov, according to his own words, already 'was under suspicion of the authorities' in connection with his enthusiasm for 'the mystical theories' of Rudolf Steiner, and the word *prana* was forced out of the language allowed by dialectical materialism. But we can easily see *prana* in 'the volitional rush of creative energy'.

Today, the effect of anthroposophy, theosophy, and the very personality of Steiner on Michael Chekhov's worldview, art, and fate is well studied. As Vladislav Ivanov writes, his enthusiasm 'was destined to grow into firm convictions constituting his life and his understanding of art'.[98] That is why it is important to emphasize that the path of the actor to his final beliefs passed through Yoga. Chekhov himself wrote in the 1950s: 'already in Moscow… I was carried away by yogis and to this day I deeply respect and value them. But, it happened that the anthroposophy of Rudolf Steiner entirely took possession of my consciousness.'[99] Although immersion in theosophy led the actor to polemics with many of the tenets

[97]   *Ibid.*, 89–90.
[98]   V. V. Ivanov, 'Introduction to "Lektsii Rudolfa Shtainera o dramaticheskom iskusstve v izlozhenii Mikhaila Chekhova. Pisma aktera k V. A. Gromovu"', *Mnemozina: Dokumenty i fakty iz istorii otechestvennogo teatra XX veka: Istoricheskii almanakh*, II, ed. by V. V. Ivanov (Moscow: Editorial URSS, 2006), 85–91.
[99]   Michael Chekhov, 'Letter to A. G. Bergstrem, May 3, 1953' in Chekhov *Literaturnoe nasledie* (1995), I, 488.

of the Yoga philosophy,[100] Chekhov repeated more than once this conclusion: it was precisely 'Yoga that step by step led me to the study of theosophy'.[101]

Thus, the philosophy and practice of Yoga, with which Chekhov first became acquainted in Stanislavsky's lessons in the First Studio, and which he developed in the process of teaching in his own Studio, exerted its influence on him.

It is interesting to compare how the newly acquired knowledge of Yoga developed in Chekhov and Vakhtangov. In contrast to Chekhov who was drawn by transcendental aspects of Yoga (it was precisely these that led him to theosophy and subsequently to anthroposophy), Vakhtangov 'utilized Yoga instrumentally with theatrical goals'.[102]

The notebook, 'Introduction to a Theoretical Course', in which young actors of Vakhtangov's Student Dramatic Studio recorded his lessons and classes, constitutes another important piece of evidence of how the introduction to Yoga in the First Studio spread beyond its confines. An entry from 15 February 1915 records Vakhtangov's words:

> by reading the philosophy of yogis it is possible to find lots of exercises. I was struck by terminology derived from it. Evidently K. S. [Stanislavsky] borrowed from there. One finds there freedom of the muscles, concentration, faith, naiveté, and justification. One finds there an exercise for developing in oneself a 'keen eye'.[103]

Vakhtangov's conclusion that completes this record explicitly explains the utilization of Yoga in the work of the Studio members: 'the goal for yogis is, of course, the perfection of man'.[104] It is for the *perfection* of the actor, i.e. of his creative apparatus, that both Stanislavsky and his students, and the

---

[100] This polemic is developed in detail in the already cited letters of Michael Chekhov to A. G. Bergstrem. See Chekhov, *Literaturnoe nasledie* (1995), I, 488–528.

[101] M. A. Chekhov, 'Zhizn i vstrechi', *Literaturnoe nasledie* (1995), I, 153.

[102] *Evgenii Vakhtangov. Dokumenty i svidetelstva*, II, 75.

[103] *Ibid.*, 73.

[104] *Ibid.*

students of his students, introduced into actor training various elements of yogic practice.

Yoga in the Opera Studio

Stanislavsky studied Yoga especially thoroughly in the process of working with actors-vocalists in the Opera Studio of the Bolshoi Theatre, work which Stanislavsky began in 1918.

As is well-known, the turning of his creative interests to opera was far from accidental. Stanislavsky was attracted to opera from early on. This interest was stoked by singing lessons that he took in his youth and later years. It is also known that he was interested in researching the work of Chaliapin, whom he considered a potential model for a dramatic actor. However, the realization of Stanislavsky's intention – to teach opera actors in a new way – coincides with his study of yogic principles of rhythmic breathing which for the yogis is the key to managing *prana*. It was also not accidental that in 1920, at the height of his interest in the connections between the rhythms of breathing and the processes of attention, interaction, and communication (and, on a broader scale, the creative sense of self on stage), arising from his work with singers, Stanislavsky made an abstract of the book by Olga Lobanova based on the principles of Yoga and titled *Breathe in the Right Way*.[105]

Thus, the realization of Stanislavsky's seriousness in the study of Yoga reveals another side of his interest in opera. We find here one of the sources of his belief in the necessity

---

[105] Vinogradskaia, *Zhizn i tvorchestvo K. S. Stanislavskogo*, III, 135. O. G. Lobanova's book, published in 1915 in Petrograd and introducing the Russian reader for the first time to the principles of the so-called three-phase breathing, has not lost its topicality even today. See O. G. Lobanova, *Dyshite pravilno: Uchenie indiiskikh iogov o dykhanii, izmenennoe Zapadom. Amerikanskaia metoda Koflera* (Moscow: Librokom, 2012). Lobanova's second book, *Pravilnoe dykhnie, rech i penie* (1923), has also been reprinted. See *Pravilnoe dykhanie Olgi Lobanovoi: Pervaia rossiiskaia dykhatelnaia praktika* (Saint Petersburg: Nevskii Prospekt, 2005).

for research on the general laws of an actor's stage existence, both in opera and in drama, and also in the fruitfulness of a joint study of actor-singers and dramatic actors.

Many talks held by Stanislavsky in the Opera Studio in 1918–1922 reveal new parallels between the System and yogic principles. They are recorded by the beginning singer Koncordia Antarova,[106] who subsequently – perhaps not by chance – was destined to engage seriously in esoteric practice and become the author of the novel *Two Lives*, which in its own right conveyed yogic wisdom.[107] In the notes of this attentive student we find, at times, a short story attributed to 'one Hindu sage' (a comparison between a non-disciplined mind and the movements of a drunk monkey),[108] and at other times, a 'Hindu proverb' (a lesson, taught to a student in reply to a question about the solution for a creative problem, urging one to rely on one's subconscious; here there arises an image frequently used by Stanislavsky of the 'pocket of the subconscious').[109] Antarova's notes were published in 1952, and there is good reason to assume that during Stanislavsky's actual lessons at the turn of the 1920s yogic terms were heard more often than in the book. However, even without using the word *prana*, Stanislavsky was able to ground the training of his actors on yogic principles. The connection with the flowing of *prana* is quite clear from the description of one of the initial exercises that involved a slow, 'breathed-through-to-the-tips-of-one's-fingers' clenching and releasing of fists (the aim

[106] Koncordia Antarova (1886–1959) – opera singer and soloist of the Bolshoi Theatre, teacher.
[107] M. Strizhenova wrote about the esoteric novel by K. E. Antarova *Two Lives* (*Dve Zhizni*), first published in 1993–94 after a long prohibition: 'As a specialist in Indian culture, I am greatly impressed by the author's subtle and deep knowledge of the peculiar life of this great Oriental country, its ancient wisdom, yoga, and venues of the secret esoteric societies of Himalayan Shambala'. See S. I. Tiuliaev, 'Konkordiia Antarova: M. Strizhenova, iz vospominanii', *Sait Lotosa. Entsiklopediia sovremennoi ezoteriki* <http://ariom.ru/wiki/KonkordijaAntarova>.
[108] K. E. Antarova, *Besedy K. S. Stanislavskogo v Studii Bolshogo teatra v 1918-1922 gg* (Moscow: Iskusstvo, 1952), 73.
[109] *Ibid.*, 100.

was to establish a link between the rhythm of breathing and one's concentration).[110] Another of Stanislavsky's demands addressed to his students has the same underlying reference to *prana*: learn to 'turn your thought into some kind of fire ball'.[111]

It was in the Opera Studio that the yogis' tenet about breathing as the foundation of life encountered Stanislavsky's belief that rhythm is the foundation of creative work in theatre. Addressing opera singers, Stanislavsky stressed:

> Music, coinciding with the rhythm of your breathing, i.e. with the basis of your whole life on Earth, should increase your concentration, bringing your whole being into harmony. Music should unite in its rhythm your thought and your feeling, and bring you into what we call true inspiration, i.e. the awakening of your intuition or subconscious.[112]

For an opera singer Stanislavsky posed the task of 'putting one's physical and psychological traits into the existing rhythm of the composer', and for a drama actor, 'to carry within oneself a composer', 'to create a rhythm for oneself', without which 'your role is nothing'.[113]

In both cases an actor's rhythm of living and, especially, the rhythm of his breathing on stage, acquire paramount importance. Stanislavsky spent a lot of time giving basic explanations of the principles of breathing, and underlined the connection between correct breathing and attention, correct breathing and the physical culture of an actor.

> With the simplest examples of physical action we need to attract his [the student's] attention to the invariable analogy: calm breathing – healthy thoughts, healthy body, healthy feelings, easy to focus attention; disturbed rhythm of breathing – always a disturbed psyche, always a sickly feeling in oneself and totally scattered attention.[114]

[110]   *Ibid.*, 73–74.
[111]   *Ibid.*, 74.
[112]   *Ibid.*
[113]   *Ibid.*
[114]   *Ibid.*, 58.

These thoughts certainly have something in common with the yogi Ramacharaka's assertion that consciousness, body, and emotions are unified by the thread of breathing and, 'in addition to physical benefit derived from correct habits of breathing, man's mental power, happiness, self-control, clear-sightedness, morals, and even his spiritual growth may be increased by an understanding of the "*Science of Breath*"'.[115]

Thus, realization of the influence of yogic practice on the Stanislavsky System sheds new light on Stanislavsky's explorations in the art of opera, and reveals one more reason for his belief in the fruitfulness of joint education of drama and opera actors. This idea will be further developed in the work of the Opera-Dramatic Studio in the middle of the 1930s.

Yoga and the Late Period of Stanislavsky's Work (1930s)

Although Stanislavsky studied and applied Yoga most fully in the first period of the development of the System, he never gave up these exercises during his lifetime. Since the term *prana* was becoming less and less ideologically acceptable, in the 1930s Stanislavsky started frequently to replace it with the word 'energy'. However, as before, in his practical work he still used the term *prana* and, more important, yogic principles themselves. For example, he did that in the production of *Boris Godunov* in the Opera Studio. According to Pavel Rumiantsev, working in November 1934 on the opera that was already running, Stanislavsky spoke a lot about the connection between an actor's plasticity and ability to make the *prana* 'flow'. Here are his remarks for the female

---

[115] Ramacharaka, *Hatha Yoga; or, The Philosophy of Physical Well-Being* (Chicago: Yogi Publication Society, 1904), 103 (hereafter referred to as Ramacharaka, *Hatha Yoga*). One can find a PDF file of this edition at https://archive.org/details/hathayoga00rama.

performer (they were rehearsing the scene between Marina Mnishek and Rangoni):

> In order to look like a tsarina I will suggest one method. There can be no half-gestures. Starting from the root of your arm (from your shoulder), you let the movement of prana (muscular energy) pass through the length of your arm. Turn your arm fully, and gradually release tension from the very tips of your fingers. Remember: fingers are of major importance! If the 'mercury'-prana will 'flow' along your hand, your legs, you will always be plastic. Dancing and gymnastics will not give plasticity as long as you do not have the inner sense of movement. It is necessary that, while you are walking, the energy streams through all of your vertebrae, and leaves through your feet. You should search for this stubbornly. Then you will be flexible... Develop your hands, fingers. Fingers are the eyes of the body... Try moving, sitting so that prana flows through your body all the time. When you walk, walk as far as the tip of your thumb. The rest of your body is totally free. Remember that the spine plays a great role in plasticity. The 'flowing of prana' should also be done in the spinal column...[116]

Citing these statements, Rumiantsev emphasizes the invariability of the yogic component in Stanislavsky's rehearsing and pedagogical practice for many years: 'These instructions reiterate, in essence, those initial exercises for developing plasticity which Stanislavsky had carried out almost fifteen years earlier with young studio members. *He constantly reiterated these demands* for all of the actors-singers, no matter what characters they embodied [italics are mine].'[117]

And at the Moscow Art Theatre's rehearsal of Bulgakov's *The Cabal of Hypocrites* on 4 May 1935, when Stanislavsky explained and showed, vividly and in detail, a typical bow of Molière's era, he stressed:

> Bear in mind that you will never succeed in making the bow unless after every movement the prana is released. Plasticity of

[116] P. I. Rumiantsev, *Stanislavskii i opera* (Moscow: Iskusstvo, 1969), 407.
[117] *Ibid.*, 407.

movement is impossible without prana. You should release all the prana without fail. […] You will draw this prana from your heart and pour this prana around.[118]

Andrew White, comparing two texts by Stanislavsky from the mid-1930s, provides the most compelling evidence that in that period the ideas of Yoga remained an integral part of the System[119]. One text is the familiar Russian edition of *An Actor's Work on Himself in the Creative Process of Experiencing*, approved for printing in 1937, and the other, the manuscript of that same book, sent to the translator Elizabeth Hapgood with the note 'the final version for America' which is now preserved in the New York Public Library for the Performing Arts. In the Russian edition, in the chapter 'Communication', we read:

How to name this invisible path and means of mutual communication? Emission of rays and reception of rays? Emanation and immanation?[120] Since we do not have any other terminology, let us settle on these words, considering that they graphically illustrate the process of communication that I am to tell you about.

The time is near when the invisible currents which are of interest to us now will be studied by science, and then a more suitable terminology will be created for them. For the present let us keep the name worked out by our actors' jargon.[121]

In the corresponding chapter of the typescript 'for America' of 1935, Stanislavsky writes more definitely:

I have read what the Hindus have to say on the topic. They believe in the existence of so-called prana, a vital energy, a force that gives life to all of our body. According to their notions, the main supply of prana is located in the solar plexus, from where it is sent throughout the entire organism.[122]

[118] K. S. Stanislavskii, *Stanislavskii repetiruet: Zapisi i stenogrammy repetitsii*, ed. by I. N. Vinogradskaia (Moscow: STD RSFSR, 1987), 427.
[119] White, 80.
[120] See footnote 20 on page 21 for different translations of Stanislavsky's term *'lucheispuskanie'*.
[121] Stanislavskii, *Ss* 9, II (1989), 338–39.
[122] K. S. Stanislavskii, 'Rabota Aktera nad Soboi, Chast' I, Okonchatel'nyi

Let us note for the future that Stanislavsky's words, cited here, are a loose quotation from Ramacharaka's book.

The comments for the third and fourth volumes of the first edition of Stanislavsky's *Collected Works* tell us that at the end of his life he rejected the concepts of *prana* and the superconscious, 'uncritically borrowed from bourgeois philosophy'[123] (here, at the same time, the French philosopher Ribot was also criticized) and, having rejected Yoga, moved on to scientific terminology and worldview. Obviously Soviet scholars were keen to prove that, following his fascination with Yoga in the practice of the System in the early period, Stanislavsky subsequently totally rejected it. However, with all the evidence above this conclusion appears to be premature.

The fact that even in 1935, twenty years after the experiments in the First Studio, Stanislavsky writes and speaks about *prana*, means that, as before, he considered a principle of Yoga a constituent part of the System and of the elements of the creative sense of self of an actor. The Memoirs of Boris Zon about Stanislavsky's rehearsals in 1933 have preserved for us additional and noteworthy evidence of that fact. The work on *The Maid of Pskov* by Rimsky-Korsakov was taking place in the Stanislavsky Opera Theatre, and Zon took notes: 'Konstantin Sergeevich made the most interesting suggestion to the performer of the role of Mikhailo. Extend your hand to Olga. Fully. So that the hand calls, *emanates* the call. (And in my direction.) Earlier we naively called that "prana".'[124]

What compelled Stanislavsky to toss this 'aside' to a young Leningrad director who was attending his rehearsals for the

dlia Ameriki' (An Actor's Work on Himself, Part I, Final Draft for America), unpublished typescript (1935), New York Public Library for the Performing Arts, Elizabeth R. Hapgood Papers, Series II: Translations, 1930–1973. Research Call Number: T-Mss 1992–039, box 7, folder 6, Chapter 10.9. See also White, 80.
[123] Stanislavskii, *Ss* 8, IV (1957), 495.
[124] K. S. Stanislavskii, *Materialy. Pis'ma. Issledovaniya* (Moscow: Akademia Nauk SSSR, 1955), 445.

first time (but attending them upon the recommendation of trusted colleagues and who was himself seriously interested in the System)? Maybe an acute need to hand over from his ceremonial confinement in Leontevskii Lane (to the outside? for posterity?) the most important information about the principles of his work?

Valerii Galendeev is right:

> On the threshold of non-existence, a man, especially a person of significance, voluntarily or involuntarily, thinks about the main thing, the thing that is demanded by the not yet exhausted spirit, and returns to his most exciting subjects. Doubly so, if these ideas and subjects have not yet been moulded into something complete and formulated, into a spiritual testament. Stanislavsky in the last years of his life, more and more, turned to the problem of *the spirituality of word, movement, and silence of an actor* [italics are mine].[125]

Galendeev connects these problems (unfortunately, without naming them directly) with yogic thoughts about the outpouring of the particles of the soul (i.e. *prana*) through the sounds of speech. But, the place in Stanislavsky's book to which he refers, is transparent: 'Do you not feel', Tortsov addresses his disciples,

> that through the vocal waves the particles of our own souls pass outside or sink inside? All these are not empty, but spiritually substantial vowel sounds, which give me the right to say, that inside, in their core, there is a piece of the human soul.[126]

According to Stanislavsky, it turns out that the atoms of speech contain, in themselves, the atoms of the human soul!

Meditating, thus, on 'the soul of sounds' and on the means of emanating it, about the plasticity of movements which 'cannot exist without prana', Stanislavsky continued – even in the twilight of his life – his dialogue with Yoga's ancient and eternal knowledge about man, about body and soul.

125   Galendeev, 105.
126   Stanislavskii, *Ss* 9, III (1990), 61.

It seems that the present overview of the use of Yoga in Stanislavsky's work is enough to draw a well-grounded conclusion about the significance of yogic theory and practice in the establishment and development of his System.

CHAPTER II

Yoga in the Literary Heritage of Stanislavsky

Understanding the constant presence of a yogic component in the practice of the System's creator, gives us a chance to reread afresh Stanislavsky's principal books and to find a yogic 'background' in his literary legacy. Many of his works, for instance, *An Actor's Work on Himself in the Creative Process of Experiencing*, contain no mention of Yoga, but we can see that many of Stanislavsky's pages are virtually permeated with yogic ideas.

In this case, Grigorii Kristi and Vladimir Prokofev, authors of the censored commentary to volumes 3 and 4 of the first edition of Stanislavsky's *Collected Works*, help us a lot. When you read them today, at first this commentary causes vexation because of its narrow-mindedness in the vein of dialectical materialism. However, let us pay attention to the Aesopian tactics used in that part of the commentary that concerns the teaching of yogis. Having expressed the expected reservations about the fact that Stanislavsky uncritically accepted the idealistic teaching of yogis, and in later years adhered to the positions of materialism, the commentators provide us with extremely valuable information about the origins of certain parts of the manuscripts on the System, even those parts where Stanislavsky was too cautious to mention his source, the books by yogi Ramacharaka.

Let the person who has ears listen. Following the clue given by Stanislavsky's commentators, it is possible to restore the whole chain leading back from many pages of Stanislavsky through the texts of Ramacharaka to their yogic origins.

But, first of all, it is worth discussing Ramacharaka's own books.

Yoga of the Twentieth Century and its Ancient Roots

The Moscow Art Theatre Archive holds two books from Stanislavsky's private library: *Hatha Yoga: Yogic Philosophy of the Physical Well-Being of a Man*, and *Raja Yoga: The Teaching of Yogis about the Mental World of Man.*[127] Translated into Russian and published in 1909 and 1914 respectively, these books, in fact, were written not in a secluded Buddhist monastery or in the hut of a yogi-hermit in India, but in the bustling American city of Chicago in 1904 and 1906 which, after the World Parliament of Religions there in 1893, became the centre for introducing Yoga to the Western world. Their author was the American William Atkinson (1862–1932), whose name and life circumstances, thanks to his secretiveness and frequent use of pseudonyms (no less than ten!), today are mostly forgotten. But at the turn of the nineteenth century, Atkinson, an attorney, writer, tradesman, and publisher, ranked among the most influential authors of New Thought in the early years of this movement. He himself took the path of esoteric knowledge after his miraculous healing at the beginning of the 1890s. In the course of thirty years he wrote more than a hundred books, many of which were published under pseudonyms, and *Yogi Ramacharaka* is only one of them. The blurb of the Yogi Publication Society asserts that this series of books about Yoga was the result of the collaborative efforts of Atkinson and Brahmin Baba Bharata, and as a sign of respect it was attributed to the latter's guru – yogi Ramacharaka. Even the Hindu sage's dates (1799–1893) and facts of his biography were included. However, there is no evidence that Baba Bharata or Ramacharaka ever really existed. Who initiated Atkinson and whether he officially converted to Hinduism is also veiled in mystery.[128]

Nonetheless, within ten years after 1903 more than a dozen books by the author Yogi Ramacharaka came out, and to this day they are still in print both in English and in Russian, topping numerous lists of literature on yoga. In this capacity

[127] Stanislavskii, *Ss* 8, IV (1957), 496.
[128] I have not succeeded in finding any reliable academic information about the real Ramacharaka or Baba Bharata. One yoga site (Ananda's site) tells a story of an intriguing correspondence of its owner with the Yogi Publication Society in Chicago in search of documents about those two. Ironically, their answers provide even more questions. See http://users.telenet.be/ananda/ramach.htm.

they remain for many people, as for Stanislavsky a hundred years ago, an introduction to a systematic knowledge of Yoga.

The structure of classical Yoga goes back to the *Yoga Sutras* of its founder, Patanjali, written (or, to be more precise, compiled from earlier teachings and philosophically grounded) in India in the second century BCE. It consists of eight 'limbs', or steps:

- *Yama*: standards of behaviour and moral self-restraint;
- *Niyama*: a series of self-purification practices, the following of religious rules and religious instructions;
- *Asana*: poses, unifying mind and body by means of physical exercise;
- *Pranayama*: control of *prana* – life energy – through rhythmic breathing and suspension of 'the restless activities of the mind';
- *Pratyahara*: withdrawal of senses from their external objects; gives inner spiritual power, allows one to achieve mental concentration, increases will power;
- *Dharana*: focusing of attention, purposeful concentration of the mind, transitioning into meditation;
- *Dhyana*: meditation, inner activity which gradually leads to *samadhi*;
- *Samadhi*: oneness with the object of meditation, meditation on *om*, the tranquil superconscious condition of the blissful realization of one's true nature, nirvana.

Sometimes these eight limbs are divided into four lower and four upper steps, of which the lower steps correspond to Hatha Yoga, while the upper steps belong to Raja Yoga. Thus, the goal of practising Hatha Yoga can be seen as thorough development of the body ensuring the meditative practice of Raja Yoga.

Of course, during the centuries of its existence, the teaching of Yoga has developed and its position has undergone serious changes. There have arisen various schools whose approaches to many aspects of the theory and practice of Yoga differ importantly. Undoubtedly, placing Yoga of the late nineteenth and early twentieth century in a historical context requires a separate study. It is worth stressing that the meeting of Stanislavsky and Yoga occurred at a moment which in many ways determined the development and spread of the centuries-old teaching. The reason for this was the stormy processes launched by the industrial development of the second half of the nineteenth century, bringing with it truly tectonic shifts in geopolitics, economics, and the culture of the whole world, changes that determined a new stage in the dialogue between the East and the West.[129]

According to Maria Kapsali, 'scholars therefore draw a distinct line between pre-modern configurations of the discipline and Modern Yoga [...], a term coined by historian Elizabeth De Michelis'.[130] Modern Yoga emerged in the second half of the nineteenth century from the blending of a variety of neo-Hindu esoteric traditions and avant-garde American occultist elements,[131] which were connected with 'metaphysics or metaphysical religion'.[132] The books of Atkinson/Ramacharaka reflected these processes of the reformulating of ancient Yoga and the formation of Modern Yoga.

Modern Yoga redefined classical Yoga in three major areas. First, following the nineteenth century preference towards the mind, a dichotomy was introduced between the meditational and physical practices, the result of which was that *Raja Yoga* as the practice of meditation overshadowed in the minds of the newly initiated *Hatha Yoga* as the practice of Yoga poses. Secondly, the concept of *prana* was reformulated according to popular metaphysical beliefs and became equated with the

---

[129] In order to appreciate the scale of these shifts in the 1860s, see the following list of the major historical events fitting into one decade: 1857–59, War of Indian Independence (Sepoy Mutiny); 1861, abolition of serfdom in Russia; 1865, abolition of slavery in the USA; 1868–89, Meiji Revolution in Japan.

[130] Maria Kapsali, 'The Presence of Yoga in Stanislavski's Work and Nineteenth Century Metaphysical Thought', 141.

[131] See Elizabeth De Michelis, 'Modern Yoga: History and Forms' in *Yoga in the Modern World: Contemporary Perspectives*, ed. by M. Singleton and J. Byrne (Oxon: Routledge, 2008), 18.

[132] Catherine Albanese, *A Republic of Mind and Spirit* (New Haven: Yale University Press, 2007), 4.

concepts of 'the vital force' and 'the fluid of life'.[133] Finally, *samadhi*, achieved in the final stage of Yoga practice, a state of unconditional freedom whereby the spirit transcends and is no longer related to matter, was translated into the language of metaphysical thought, and as such denotes 'access to higher or "superconscious" states'[134] and 'the subsequent forging of the individual with the collective mind'.[135]

In this way, Kapsali – who correctly indicated the necessity of analyzing the influence on Stanislavsky of Yoga not in general, but of the Yoga of a concrete historical period – concludes:

> Through the development of the *'prana'* and *'samadhi* model', spiritual development is divorced from the supernatural achievements of Tantric doctrines and/or the divine grace of orthodox Hinduism. Rather, spiritual ascendance becomes democratized and subjected to laws, which can be discovered and followed by the aspirant. In such a manner, yoga acquires a prescriptive and predictable character, since it becomes the answer to a – predominantly American – nineteenth-century pervasive desire for a *technique* that could place both otherworldly attainment as well as worldly success within everyone's reach.[136]

In a sense, it was lucky that Stanislavsky's introduction to the ideas of Yoga – at the moment when he was also seeking for *technique*, but for an actor – occurred through the books of Atkinson/Ramacharaka.

---

[133]   See Elizabeth De Michelis, *A History of Modern Yoga* (New York: Continuum, 2004), 161–64.

[134]   De Michelis, 153.

[135]   Kapsali, 142.

[136]   *Ibid.* Kapsali's article poses the question as to the correlation and sources of influence on Stanislavsky's work and argues that it was not Yoga, but nineteenth-century metaphysical thought – through Modern Yoga – that was of paramount importance. However, taking into account that her discussion is about the interaction of the philosophical thought of the East and of the West, it is difficult not to recall the harmonious image of yin-yang. It seems it is more productive not to contrast the cultures, but to emphasize the integrity and productiveness of the influence on the Stanislavsky System of knowledge drawn from the books of the American William Walker Atkinson aka Yogi Ramacharaka.

There is no doubt that this interpretation of Yoga was adapted for the understanding of Western readers. It is they whom the American yogi addresses, freely quoting European and American scholars of the nineteenth and twentieth centuries and intentionally not overburdening the readers with the specifics of separate branches and schools of Hindu Yoga. Atkinson lays out a kind of generalized yogic tradition, and 'does not favour one specific school or philosophy of Yoga, as an actual Yogi might'.[137]

Sharon Carnicke correctly observes that when Jerzy Grotowski, following in Stanislavsky's footsteps, tried to apply Yoga to theatrical work on the basis of *genuine* Hindu texts, he found himself in a dead end. After all, the goal of practising Yoga is liberation from the wheel of suffering, leaving behind reactions to the surrounding earthly life and moving into the eternal absolute. Naturally, at a certain stage this started to contradict the aim of theatre and theatrical expressiveness. Grotowski wrote:

> we began by doing yoga directed toward absolute concentration. Is it true, we asked, that yoga can give actors the power of concentration? We observed that despite all our hopes the opposite happened. There was a certain concentration, but it was introverted. This concentration destroys all expression; it's an internal sleep, an inexpressive equilibrium: a great rest which ends all actions. This should have been obvious because the goal of yoga is to stop three processes: thought, breathing, and ejaculation. That means all life processes are stopped and one finds fullness and fulfillment in conscious death, autonomy enclosed in our own kernel.[138]

It was easier for Stanislavsky to master Yoga: introducing Western readers to the world of Eastern wisdom, Ramacharaka laid out Yoga principles as the basis for the ability to control oneself, as the art of self-improvement, without accentuating the true end objective of reaching nirvana. Although

---

[137]   White, 82.
[138]   Jerzy Grotowski, *Towards a Poor Theatre* (New York: Simon and Schuster, 1968), 252.

Ramacharaka saw Yoga as a means of turning consciousness inward into oneself, which contradicted the basic creative task of the System, namely to find the means to express externally the feeling experienced internally, Stanislavsky was able to adapt the yogic idea of 'disengaging oneself from distracting impressions' into the fruitful condition of concentration and attention during a performance. The System's creator knew that for an actor the main 'distracting impression', with which he fought so passionately, is the frightening black hole of the auditorium. In this sense existence behind the famous 'fourth wall' seems related to the yogic disengagement from the temptations of the world.

At the same time Stanislavsky completely understood the difference between his practical tasks and the end objectives of Yoga. During lectures in November 1919 for the actors of the Moscow Art Theatre, he stressed: 'It turns out that a thousand years ago they [yogis] were searching for the very same things that we are searching for, however, we move into art, and they, into their afterworld'.[139]

Let us once again turn to the notes of Stanislavsky's classes in the Opera Studio. In his discussions, Stanislavsky guides the students through 'general for all of them, *steps of creation* [italics are mine], no matter what the epochs and individualities of the people are',[140] and these steps which 'everyone who has dedicated his or her life to the art of the stage' should ascend are closer to the stages of esoteric moral self-improvement than to the set of narrowly professional demands.[141]

The first step is concentration; the second, vigilance; the third, fearlessness, courage in creation; the fourth, creative tranquillity. Similar to the transition to elevated matters of Raja Yoga after the first four limbs of Hatha Yoga, after the four steps of an actor's work that establishes the unity of the

---

[139] Cited in O. A. Radischeva, *Stanislavskii i Nemirovich-Danchenko: Istoriia teatralnykh otnoshenii, 1917–1938* (Moscow: Akter. Regisser. Teatr, 1999), 61.
[140] Antarova, 79.
[141] *Ibid.*

actor with himself, Stanislavsky designates lofty artistic goals. Upward movement continues through the fifth step: 'bringing all the powers of one's feelings and thoughts, recast into physical action, to the greatest tension', 'to the precision of *heroic tension*'.[142]

The sixth step is connected to cultivating an actor's charm on stage, the nobleness with which he refines the passions he portrays.[143] Here, completely in the spirit of Buddhism, Stanislavsky speaks about 'the fatal moments when the human spirit seeks *to liberate* itself from passion'.[144]

Finally, 'the last step without which one does not live in art. *It is joy.*'[145] This striving for the joy of creative work as the crown of actor training contains the most significant lesson for future generations and the essence of Stanislavsky's ethical position. His famous words, written on the day of his seventieth birthday, confirm that the creator of the System himself, having gone through all of the above-mentioned steps in Salieri's tormenting manner of self-searching, savoured the happiness of the seventh step in full:

> I have lived a long life. I have seen a lot. I was rich. Then I grew poor. I have seen the world. I had a good family, children. Life has scattered them across the world. I sought fame. I found it. I saw laurels, I was young. I have grown old. Soon it will be time to die.
>
> Now ask me: what constitutes happiness on Earth?
>
> It is in the cognitive process. It is in art and work, in coming to know art.
>
> Getting to know art in oneself, you come to know nature, the life of the world, the meaning of life, you get to know the soul – talent.
>
> There is no happiness greater than that.[146]

Probably, it is not an accident that the arithmetic number of steps in Yoga does not coincide with that in Stanislavsky's descriptions of an actor's steps in mastering himself. After all,

---

[142]   *Ibid.*, 90–91.
[143]   *Ibid.*, 94.
[144]   *Ibid.*, 96.
[145]   *Ibid.*
[146]   Stanislavskii, *Ss* 8, VIII (1961), 324–25.

the eighth step of Yoga leads to nirvana, and here is where the end objectives of Yoga and of an actor's creative work, and hence of the System, diverge definitively.

Therefore, the utilization of Yoga for theatrical goals required definite reorientation. After Stanislavsky, this problem was most fully interpreted in the practice of Jerzy Grotowski. The above-mentioned difficulties in his adaptation of classical Yoga for theatre did not lead to a loss of interest on the part of the Polish director. Moreover, in contrast to many (including Stanislavsky), Grotowski was interested in Yoga not only in connection with its potential possibilities for training theatre actors. Yoga interested Grotowski outside of its theatrical utilization; if one can say so, it interested him 'before' theatre.[147] And, 'after' theatre. Passion for Yoga and the study of it preceded Grotowski's ardour for the theatre, and his departure from traditional theatre to realize his predestined path of cognition, highlights this initial position of the director-thinker. After all, theatre for Grotowski was only a means, not an end, and as Richard Schechner justly states, his 'goal was not political, as with Brecht; nor artistic, as with Stanislavsky; nor revolutionary, as with Artaud.

---

[147]   Paul Brunton's *A Search in Secret India* (London: Rider & Co., 1934), which Grotowski read in his childhood, greatly impressed him. According to Osiński, 'It is not an exaggeration to state that Brunton's book accompanied Grotowski for his entire life' (Zbigniew Osiński, *Jerzy Grotowski's Journeys to the East* [London and New York: Icarus and Routledge, 2014], 69). Eugenio Barba also states that even in the 1990s Grotowski 'still considered Maharshi to be his spiritual master, that he had copies of Brunton's book in English, French, Italian and Polish, and that he made everyone who worked with him read the chapter about Maharshi' (*Land of Ashes and Diamonds* [Aberystwyth: Black Mountain Press, 1999], 140). Barba's book lists the series of Hindu themes discussed by the two men of theatre (ibid., 48–50). Among other books important for Grotowski were: Romain Rolland, *The Life of Ramakrishna* (Calcutta: Asvaita Ashrama, 1934); Mircea Eliade, *Yoga: Essai sur l'origine de la mystique Indienne* (Paris: Bucuresti, 1936). In English: Mircea Eliade, *Yoga: Immortality and Freedom* (Princeton: Princeton University Press, 1969). It is my pleasure to thank Zbigniew Osiński for his kind sharing of his unpublished manuscript with me, and I extend my gratitude to Eugenio Barba, who presented his book to me with a lovely inscription, rather meaningful to the theme of my book: 'To Sergei with whom I share the panreligious cult of Stanislavski and his loyal and heretic heir. In friendship. E. Barba. Holstebro. 6.05.2013.'

Grotowski's goal was spiritual: the search for and education of each performer's soul'.[148]

A deep knowledge of Yoga, a comparison of texts, either linked to ancient traditions or reinterpreted (the teaching of Ramana Maharshi[149] and Ramakrishna[150]), and contemporary interpretations of Yoga (the asanas of B. K. S. Iyengar[151]) helped Grotowski realize a principal improvement in the utilization of Yoga and, in his own words, to 'change all the currents'.[152] Demonstrating together with Ryszard Cieślak in 1966 the 'training and drill' of the Theatre Laboratory, many of whose exercises were based on the principles of Yoga, Grotowski commented that: 'The essential difference between these exercises and Yoga is that these [exercises of Cieślak] are dynamic exercises aimed at the exterior. This exteriorization replaces the introversion typical of Yoga.'[153]

It is worth noting that the paragraph cited on page 60 of this book from *Towards a Poor Theatre* ends with Grotowski's

[148]   Richard Schechner, 'Exoduction', *The Grotowski Sourcebook*, ed. by Liza Wolford and Richard Schechner (London: Routledge, 1997), 475.
[149]   Ramana Maharshi (1879–1950) – an Indian guru. Since the 1930s his teachings have been popularized in the West. Burton's book that so impressed young Grotowski was of importance in that process. Grotowski visited the shrine of Maharshi at Tiruvannaamalai during his 1969 trip to India. For his own detailed account of that see Zbigniew Raszewski, *Raptularz* (Diary), ed. by Edyta and Tomasz Kubikowscy (London: Puls, 2004), vol. 1, 484–88. Cited in Osiński, 66.
[150]   Ramakrishna Paramahamsa (1836–1886) – an Indian guru, reformer of Hinduism, mystic, preacher. His religious school of thought led to the formation of the Ramakrishna Mission by his chief disciple Swami Vivekananda. Grotowski visited the shrine of Ramakrishna during his 1969 trip to India (See Jerzy Grotowski, 'Letter to Eugenio Barba, August 10, 1969' in Eugenio Barba, *Land of Ashes and Diamonds* [Aberystwyth: Black Mountain Press, 1999], 169). Barba also claims: 'Hinduism was our privileged point of encounter. Ramana Maharshi […] had played an important part in the life of Grotowski, and Ramakrishna in mine.' (Barba, 48).
[151]   Bellur Krishnamukar Sundara Iyengar (1918–2014) was one of the most outstanding contemporary masters of yoga, the founder of Iyengar Yoga, the author of numerous books and fundamental texts on yoga. In 2004, according to the American magazine *Time*, Iyengar entered the list of the hundred most influential people on the planet. See B. K. S. Iyengar, *Light on Yoga* (New York: Schocken, 1966).
[152]   Jerzy Grotowski, *Towards a Poor Theatre* (New York: Simon and Schuster, 1968), 252.
[153]   *Ibid.*, 186.

conclusion: 'I don't attack it [Yoga] but it's not for actors.'[154] Taken out of context, this sentence brings many researchers to the claim that Grotowski refused the use of Yoga in his theatrical practice. The erroneousness of this opinion becomes evident from both an analysis of videotapes of the actor training and performances of the Theatre Laboratory and from a more careful reading of Grotowski's book. Indeed, literally the next paragraph speaks of the senselessness of a repudiation of Yoga. Grotowski sets a task of 'change[-ing] all their currents', i.e. transferring the emphasis, when using Yoga in actor training, from an introverted immersion in oneself to communication with one's partner.[155]

The remark by Grotowski about what precisely drew him to the practices of the Hindu yogi is characteristic. In a letter to Eugenio Barba from India where Grotowski was travelling in 1969, he wrote:

> I also met the most important Baul master (Yoga through song and dance),[156] who devotes himself to many of the same things as I do – the anatomy of the actor. *It is amazing to see how certain aspects of the craft are objective* [italics are mine].[157]

This search for the *objective* laws of the actor's craft is definitely common for both Stanislavsky's and Grotowski's exploration of Yoga.

However, an analysis of Yoga's influence on Grotowski – who, in choosing a future profession vacillated among Oriental studies, psychiatry, and directing, and who stated that he 'began where Stanislavsky finished', whose appearance after his pilgrimage to India in 1970 changed so dramatically that he was not recognized, not only by his actors but even by his own brother, and who, at the end of his life, wanted his ashes to be scattered over India which was both far and close

---

[154] *Ibid.*, 252.
[155] *Ibid.*
[156] The Bauls are members of a Bengali mystical, esoteric sect, most of whom are begging, wandering minstrels.
[157] Jerzy Grotowski, 'Letter to Eugenio Barba, August 10, 1969' in Barba, 169.

to him[158] – is the subject of separate research.[159] Nevertheless, how the secular reorientation ('change of the current') of yoga was possible becomes clear if you just imagine how many people in the world today engage in modified versions of Hatha Yoga and meditation, mostly in order to maintain their physical shape and to get rid of stress.

This same kind of reorientation of the yogic techniques directed inwards and upwards, but for the aims of actor training, was performed by Stanislavsky in earlier years. However, among his numerous notes in the copy of *Hatha Yoga* preserved in the archive of the Moscow Art Theatre, there is a marked paragraph containing a warning for those who regard Yoga only as a set of physical stunts or just an Eastern form of physical culture. It seems that Stanislavsky understood well that the most valuable thing in Yoga for acting was the deep connection between outward physical exercises and spiritual education, the multi-sidedness of the continuous chain of exercises, permeated by an ascending line of self-improvement. This zeal for continuous apprenticeship is, of course, central to Stanislavsky. That is why he thoroughly studied both *Hatha Yoga* and *Raja Yoga* by Ramacharaka, and it was from these books that he drew many of the most important tenets of the System.

It is interesting to place these books beside the volumes of Stanislavsky's *Collected Works* and to compare them carefully. What follows develops from the train of thought of Sharon Carnicke, who as far as I am aware, was the first to make an attempt at textual comparison of the works of Stanislavsky and Ramacharaka.[160]

---

[158]   See Zbigniew Osiński, *Jerzy Grotowski's Journeys to the East* (Holstebro, Malta, Wrocław, London and New York: Icarus and Routledge, 2014), 74; N. Z. Bashindzhagian, *Kontury biografii: Ezhi Grotovskii. Ot Bednogo teatra k Iskusstvu-provodniku* (Moscow: Akter. Regisser. Teatr, 2003), 24.

[159]   This theme is developed in more detail in Kapsali, 'The Use of Yoga in Actor Training and Theatre Making', 84–99; Osiński, 55–91; and Maria Kapsali '"I don't attack it but it's not for actors": the use of yoga by Jerzy Grotowski', *Theatre, Dance and Performance Training*, 1 (2) (2010), 185–98.

[160]   Carnicke, 172–74.

A Comparative Reading of Stanislavsky and Ramacharaka

We already cited the words of Vakhtangov accompanying his reading of yogic literature and reflecting the joy of recognizing the familiar vocabulary of the Stanislavsky System: 'The terms taken from there [i.e. 'the philosophy of Yoga'] struck me. Evidently K. S. [Stanislavsky] borrowed from there.'[161] But it turns out that not only the terms, but also many of the images of the System find their direct analogy in the texts of the American yogi.

For example, both authors, Ramacharaka and Stanislavsky, call the subconscious their 'friend' who helps in one's mental and creative work.[162] Both of them surprise the reader with the fact that the subconscious occupies 90% of our mental life. While doing this, Stanislavsky, without citing the source, borrows verbatim from Ramacharaka the references to the psychologists Elmar Götz and Henry Maudsley.[163] For both, the essence of education and training is in the ability to use, in Ramacharaka's words, 'the subconscious mind under orders of the conscious mind',[164] or, according to Stanislavsky, 'the work of the subconscious sphere of thinking, under the command of the conscious sphere'.[165] Both describe memory as 'the storehouse' from which the particles of human experience are retrieved.[166] Finally, they are similar in their striving to grasp the truth in a new way: 'not as it had appeared before, imperfectly and erroneously',[167] and in the understanding that 'life's truth on stage is not at all what exists in reality'.[168]

[161] *Vakhtangov: Dokumenty*, II, 73.

[162] Stanislavskii, *Ss* 9, II (1989), 436; Ramacharaka. *A Series of Lessons in Raja Yoga* (Chicago: The Yogi Publication Society, 1906), 235 (hereafter referred to as Ramacharaka, *Raja Yoga*). One can find a PDF file of this edition at https://archive.org/details/seriesoflessonsi00rama.

[163] Stanislavskii, *Ss* 9, IV (1991), 140; Ramacharaka, *Raja Yoga*, 149.

[164] Ramacharaka, *Raja Yoga*, 224.

[165] Stanislavskii, *Ss* 9, II (1989), 61, 427, 437.

[166] *Ibid*., 290; Ramacharaka, *Raja Yoga*, 25, 53, 132, etc.

[167] Ramacharaka, *Raja Yoga*, 81.

[168] Stanislavskii, *Ss* 9, IV (1991), 380.

Reading Ramacharaka's books today, one comes across numerous phrases, images, and keywords well-known from Stanislavsky. Moreover, Ramacharaka's works 'clearly provided Stanislavsky with more than conceptual notions and practical exercises; they provided a structural model for what he most passionately wanted: to assist actors in harnessing the creative state'.[169] Overall, the Stanislavsky System teaches mastery of the creative state by the same means as 'the Science of Raja Yoga teaches, as its basic principle, the Control of the Mind'.[170]

Ramacharaka proposes a consecutive programme which, like the books on the System, develops from spiritual work on oneself to physical exterior work. Both systems of training are based on the fact that 'before man attempts to solve the secrets of the Universe without, he should master the Universe within – the Kingdom of the Self'.[171]

This knowledge about oneself should be achieved on the level of feelings. Ramacharaka emphasizes: 'The Yogi Masters are not satisfied if the Candidate forms merely a clear intellectual conception of this Actual Identity, but they insist that he must *feel* the truth of the same – must become aware of the Real Self.'[172] And with the words that are very much common to all the future readers of the System, the American yogi states that 'Truth is not truth to you until you have proven it in your own *experience* [italics are mine]'.[173] This is where Stanislavsky's famous, oft-repeated tenet comes from: 'in our lore, to understand means to feel'.[174]

Even the titles of the System's books reflect this same yogic sequence of self-improvement from the internal to the external:

---

[169] Carnicke, 173.
[170] Ramacharaka, *Raja Yoga*, 79.
[171] *Ibid.*, 1.
[172] *Ibid.*, v.
[173] *Ibid.*, 40.
[174] Stanislavskii, *Ss* 9, I (1988), 373. To underline the polyphony of influences on Stanislavsky it is worth mentioning that this statement also appeared in Sergei Volkonsky's books on voice and speech.

an actor's work on oneself (first in the process of 'experiencing', and only after that, in the process of 'embodiment'), then an actor's work on the role. One encounters even the crucially important word 'work' in all of Ramacharaka's writings. He instructs his students: 'Do not forget that all that we know we have "worked for". There is nothing that comes to the idler, or shirker.'[175]

Of course, this way of putting the matter is very important to the founder of the first art theatre in Russia, which was established as a challenge to the private companies with low standards; it was created out of his wish 'to cleanse art from any kind of filth, to build a temple instead of a fairground booth'.[176] Not by accident the necessity for creative discipline was stressed in both the practical life of the Moscow Art Theatre and in its studios of all periods, and in the literary works on the System. 'I consider myself obliged to be strict during collective work as if we were in the military', declared the kindest Rakhmanov/Suler, the assistant of Tortsov/Stanislavsky.[177]

Among other of Ramacharaka's terms which are echoed in the Stanislavsky System we can mention 'task (*zadacha*)'.[178] Yogis also based their work on 'spiritual tasks'.

Besides that, Ramacharaka sets forth in *Raja Yoga* a system of 'exercises or development drills'.[179] Stanislavsky creates a System that includes 'training and drill'. Ramacharaka shows his students the *Path*, Stanislavsky stresses that 'the System is a guide'.[180] Immersion in 'the object of the examination and consideration',[181] which Ramacharaka considered crucial for successful concentration, was echoed in an actor's arsenal

[175] Ramacharaka, *Raja Yoga*, 126.
[176] Stanislavskii, *Ss* 9, I (1988), 268.
[177] Stanislavskii, *Ss* 9, II (1989), 48.
[178] 'Task' (*zadacha*) – Hapgood (1936) translates this term of the Stanislavsky System as 'objective'; Benedetti (2008) translates it as 'task'. It has also been translated as 'task/problem' (Carnicke).
[179] Ramacharaka. *Raja Yoga*, 8.
[180] Stanislavskii, *Ss* 9, III (1990), 371.
[181] Ramacharaka, *Raja Yoga*, 33–34.

as 'objects of attention'. One can more easily assimilate the thoughts of a person, as well as of a play, when they are divided into 'pieces' or 'bits'.[182] Just as a tree growing in a crevice adjusts its form to the available space through the yogic 'principle of adaptation', so actors use 'adaptations' in the given circumstances of a play and of the production.

According to both Ramacharaka and Stanislavsky, if one's 'wishing'[183] or 'want'[184] is not strong enough, neither man nor character will reach his goal.

We can find more and more examples of Stanislavsky's and Ramacharaka's positions coinciding. What is of paramount importance is that both Ramacharaka and Stanislavsky present their systems as open ones, as 'guides', not as hard and fast rules. Both teachers offer their students various paths to follow.

Various paths to follow! – this diversity of the System's approaches is something to be remembered by today's theatre practitioners and scholars. It is well known that in the 1930s Stanislavsky's research interests were mostly connected with the development of action-based approaches in actor training (that later were shaped in the Method of Psycho-Physical Actions and Action Analysis). It is often forgotten that even at that time Stanislavsky never rejected the use of affective memory. However, in a letter written by Stanislavsky in 1937 to his American translator Elizabeth Hapgood he stated clearly:

> This is untrue and complete nonsense that I renounced memory of feelings. I repeat: it is the main element in our creative work. I had to renounce only the name (affective) and to recognize more than previously the significance of memory, which feeling suggests to us, i.e. that on which our art is based.[185]

---

[182]   'Bit' (*kusok*) – Hapgood (1936) translates this term of the Stanislavsky System as 'unit'; Benedetti (2008) translates it as 'bit'. In the lessons of Russian émigré teachers, American students heard this word as 'beat'; thus, it often became 'beats' in US usage.
[183]   Ramacharaka, *Raja Yoga*, 24.
[184]   Stanislavskii, *Ss* 9, II (1989), 220, 221, etc. 'Want' (*khotenie*) might also be translated as 'desire'.
[185]   Stanislavskii, *Ss* 9, IX (1999), 665.

Moreover, in his discussion with the graduating students of the Director's Department of GITIS on 15 May 1938, Stanislavsky said that 'One must offer actors different paths. One of these is the path of action. There is also another path: you can go from feeling towards action, actuating feeling first.'[186] This tolerance of Stanislavsky towards the diversity of approaches to the creative state of mind and body is something that his followers were prone to underestimate.

Stanislavsky's thoughts, expressed three months before his death, are probably not just 'modeling himself on Yogi teachers' as Carnicke puts it,[187] or copying the tenets of Ramacharaka's books that he read two decades earlier. Rather, Stanislavsky was drawing conclusions from extensive research that included dialogue with numerous sources, among which Yoga was one of the most important, but not the only one. The main thing is that in these final years, Stanislavsky approached overcoming the dichotomies characteristic of the Western mind and gave preference to the method of etudes in which analysis and embodiment, the internal and the external, the psychic and the physical of the actor-creator, merge holistically.

Of course, Ramacharaka's books were not the only source of information about Yoga and esoteric teachings for Stanislavsky. In 1916 the Moscow Art Theatre started working on the production of the play *The King of the Dark Chamber* by the 1913 Nobel Prize winner, Bengali author Rabindranath Tagore. At the centre of this dramatic allegory about spiritual enlightenment there is the image of an enigmatically mystical king who appears to his subjects always under the veil of darkness, and they can only guess about his true essence, only believe in his existence.

Stanislavsky spoke enthusiastically about the play. He saw in the production of 'a deep religious miracle play' possibilities to widen the range of theatre and the acting skill

[186]   *Stanislavskii repetiruet*, 565.
[187]   Carnicke, 173.

of actors. 'Rabindranath, Aeschylus – these are the real ones. We cannot play that, but we should at least try. The authors will help', he wrote to Vladimir Nemirovich-Danchenko.[188] Although the production never opened (rehearsals ended with the performance of fragments of the production in December 1918), the work on this material widened Stanislavsky's knowledge about Hinduism and the spiritual values of the East. During work on the production, lectures on Hindu philosophy were organized. This knowledge seemed necessary to Stanislavsky for practical work even outside the Tagore project and in March 1919 in the discussion with the Moscow Art Theatre actors about new theatrical forms, he advised that they invite 'the Hindu Suhrawardy' again in order to continue their conversation.[189]

Nevertheless, Stanislavsky's main source of studying Yoga were Ramacharaka's books, and that is why it was important to concentrate mostly on a comparison between the American yogi's works and those of the author of the System.

The study of the basics of the ancient Hindu teaching about man, having begun for Stanislavsky in that very same 1911 when the System was declared the official method of work of the Moscow Art Theatre, turned out to be not just 'another infatuation of Konstantin Sergeevich'. It took the form of a long-term and fertile influence of Yoga on Stanislavky's searches and those of his students. Many generations of

---

[188]   Stanislavskii, Ss 9, VIII (1998), 449.
[189]   Stanislavskii, Ss 9, VI (1994), 488. Shahid Suhrawardy (1890–1965) was a Pakistani poet, historian, diplomat and, in the words of V. A. Maksimova 'one of the most original and little known figures of the Moscow Art Theatre's entourage', Mnemozina, 180. He collaborated with the Moscow Art Theatre and with its Prague group (he directed the interludes by Cervantes in which Stanislavsky's son Igor Alekseev played; later he helped Vasilii Kachalov with the revival of Hamlet). He was especially close with Maria Germanova; together they staged the revival of The King of the Dark Chamber in Berlin (1922), and then he lived in her apartment in Paris for several years. (Germanova in her turn was in India in the 1930s at the invitation of Suhrawardy and there, with his influence, became good friends with Nikolai Roerich and became carried away with Buddhism.) In 1954, Suhrawardy was the ambassador of Pakistan to Spain and the Vatican. See also Shverubovich, 279–80.

actors during Stanislavsky's life – actors of the First Studio in the 1910s, singers of the Opera Studio in the 1920s, and students of the Opera-Dramatic Studio in the 1930s – went through the exercises of the System based on Yoga. Many generations of actors after Stanislavsky, carrying out their everyday preparations (whenever they are called 'training and drill' or actor's 'toilet' or just *trening*) according to the System, paid tribute to yogic principles, sometimes – thanks to the politics of Soviet censorship in the field of art and culture – without even realizing it. Rephrasing Lev Dodin, who said that 'when an actor performs in the right way, he performs according to Stanislavsky, even if he does not like Stanislavsky',[190] we can claim that when an actor does *trening* according to the Stanislavsky System, he depends upon the centuries-old experience of Yoga, even if he has never practised Yoga.

A parallel reading of the texts by Ramacharaka and Stanislavsky also gives us the possibility to consider in a new way the elements of an actor's creative sense of self, i.e. the elements of the Stanislavsky System which are directly connected to the teaching of Yoga. Among them are muscle relaxation, communication, emission of rays and reception of rays, attention, and mental images, or visualizations.[191] Special attention should be paid to Stanislavsky's views on the structure of the unconscious activity of a person, including his subconscious and superconscious. It is from *Raja Yoga* that Stanislavsky had the idea of the connection between the creative state and the unconscious state, thus borrowing the notion of the superconscious as the source of inspiration, of creative intuition and of transcendental knowledge. In the introduction to *An Actor's Work on Himself*, Stanislavsky points to the key meaning of the chapter 'The Subconscious

---

[190]   L. A. Dodin, 'Chelovek – sushchestvo tragicheskoe, i emu neobxodimo tragicheskoe iskusstvo: Interviu Iu. Kovalenko', *Izvestiya*, 6 May 1997.

[191]   The meanings of each of these elements of the System as well as variants of their translation are discussed and analyzed in Chapter III.

in the Creative Sense of Self of an Actor', in which for him is 'the essence of creation and of the whole System'.[192]

The third chapter of this book focuses on a detailed analysis of yogic elements in the Stanislavsky System.

[192] Stanislavskii, *Ss* 9, II (1989), 42.

Yogic Elements of
the Stanislavsky System

Let us try to compare the drawing of the System made by Stanislavsky[193] with the ancient Indian drawings depicting the location of yogic chakras (energy centres), situated along the spine of the human body. Stanislavsky's picture unintentionally resembles a human body where numerous wavy lines, changing their colours and signifying various elements of the internal and external creative sense of self of an actor, bear a resemblance to the left and right lungs of man. They are located on both sides of the vertical, the spine. In Stanislavsky's drawing this vertical is defined *as the perspective of the role – the through action.*

Three circles, three drivers of psychic life, are threaded on this vertical: *mind, will,* and *feeling.* They are depicted as circles, just like the circles signifying chakras in the yogic chart. Thus, these drivers of psychic life are clearly likened to the chakras of man and act as some kind of 'actor's chakras', the sources of an actor's energy.

It seems that the graphics of this diagram are deliberate for Stanislavsky. The similarity to the human organism was meant to suggest the foundation in natural science of the elements of the System, i.e. the laws of life, the laws of the organic nature of the human being/actor.

It should be remembered that Stanislavsky became acquainted with Ramacharaka's books during the analytical period of the creation of the System, when he apparently was collecting the objectively existing elements of the creative sense of self, the laws describing the natural functioning of the human organism. In the manuscript 'The Programme of an Article: My System' (1909), that very piece where the term *System* appears in Stanislavsky's work for the first time, among the elements necessary for a genuine creative sense of self the following are mentioned: *muscle relaxation and muscle tension, communication, creative concentration or the*

[193]   Stanislavskii, *Ss* 8, III (1955), 360.

circle of concentration.[194] Yoga gave Stanislavsky concrete techniques for developing these qualities of an actor.

Let us look at the basic elements of the System, on whose formation Yoga had an essential influence, and proceed in the order of an ascending path of self-improvement, as suggested by classical Yoga with its eight steps.

It makes sense to start with *Hatha Yoga* where Ramacharaka, without touching on the first two steps, *yama* and *niyama*, lays out the third and fourth steps of classical Yoga: *asana* – the science of uniting mind and body through physical exercise, and *pranayama* – the skills of controlling *prana* through rhythmic breathing. From here Stanislavsky borrowed the technique of relaxation, muscle relaxation, and, as was already noted in the analysis of Stanislavsky's work in the Opera Studio, the technique and principles of rhythmic breathing.[195]

Relaxation of Muscles (Muscular Release)[196]

Stanislavsky believed that the first step on the path to achieving a creative sense of self was the removal of muscular tension, and although he did not practise asanas, i.e. the poses of Yoga (Ramacharaka does not describe them directly either), he paid much attention to developing skills of physical relaxation.

In Chapter XXII, 'Science of Relaxation', Ramacharaka says that 'The Hatha Yogi gurus, when teaching the lesson of

[194] K. S. Stanislavskii, 'Programme of the Article: My System, June, 1909' (unpublished document from the Archive of the Museum of the Moscow Art Theatre), K. S. Stanislavsky Collection, no. 628, 46–48. Also see G. V. Kristi, 'Kniga K. S. Stanislavskogo "Rabota aktera nad soboi"' in *Ss* 8, II (1954), xviii.
[195] For information on how these principles are used today see the following workbook: E. I. Chernaia, *Vospitanie fonatsionnogo dykhaniia s ispolzovaniem printsipov dykhatelnoi gimnastiki 'iogi'*.
[196] 'Relaxation of Muscles' (*Osvobozhdenie myshts*) – Hapgood (1936) translates this term of the Stanislavsky System as 'relaxation of muscles'; Benedetti (2008) translates it as 'muscular release'. It has also been translated as 'relaxation' (Carnicke).

Relaxation, often direct their student's attention to the cat, or animals of the cat-tribe, the panther or leopard [...]'.[197] This pedagogical approach was picked up by Stanislavsky. Thus, in the chapter 'Relaxation of Muscles' in *An Actor's Work on Himself in the Creative Process of Experiencing*, a domestic cat becomes the principal teacher of the student Nazvanov,[198] who was injured in a class presentation as a result of muscle tension, and had to miss Tortsov's lessons. Tortsov's assistant, Rakhmanov (Sulerzhitsky's alter ego), who visits Nazvanov, instructs him in the following way:

> 'The Hindus teach, my dear, that we should lie in the same manner as little children and animals lie. As animals!', he repeated for persuasiveness. 'Be sure of that!'
>
> Further, Ivan Platonovich [Rakhmanov] explained why that is necessary. It turns out that if you put a child or a cat on the sand, let them relax or fall asleep, and then carefully lift them, an imprint of the whole body will be left on the sand. If you do the same experiment with an adult, the only imprint will be that of the strongly pressed shoulder blades and sacrum because the other parts of the body, due to constant, chronic, habitual muscle tension, will touch the sand more weakly, and therefore will not leave an imprint.
>
> In order to lie like children and leave an imprint on a soft soil, you have to completely release all your muscle tension. Such a condition allows the body to rest in the best possible way. A half hour or an hour of such rest is more refreshing than a whole night of sleep. It is not for nothing that caravan leaders resort to such methods. They cannot linger too long in the desert, so they have to reduce their sleep to a minimum. The reduction in sleep time is compensated by complete release of the body from muscle tension which revitalizes the tired body.[199]

In Chapter XXIII of *Hatha Yoga*, titled 'Rules for Relaxation', Ramacharaka presents a whole series of 'loosening up

---

[197] Ramacharaka, *Hatha Yoga*, 175.
[198] In the English translations of Stanislavsky's books, the student Nazvanov who is making notes in Tortsov's classes on acting in the form of a diary is usually referred to as Kostya.
[199] Stanislavskii, *Ss* 9, II (1989), 190.

exercises' after which he moves on to stretching exercises, mind relaxation exercises, and the exercise 'a moment's rest'.[200] There are a lot of examples of this type of exercise in Stanislavsky as well. At the same time it should be noted that these exercises are presented in quite a general form. This part of the System remains one of the most unfinished and open, calling for development and allowing for a welcome addition of the most diverse methods, both yogic and completely different. Therefore, it is not surprising that in the part of modern actor training intended to free muscle tension, more and more exercises are added to the original set of exercises, some of them coming from Eastern martial arts, others from bioenergetics, from medical gymnastics, etc.

It is necessary also to pay special attention, as Kapsali does,[201] to where the chapter 'Relaxation of Muscles' appears in Stanislavsky's book. In keeping with its content, it should belong to the second volume of *An Actor's Work* (titled *An Actor's Work on Himself in the Creative Process of Embodiment*), devoted to the external technique of an actor. After all, even formally the discussion in this chapter is about the body, about muscles. Nevertheless, it is placed by Stanislavsky in the first volume of *An Actor's Work* (titled *An Actor's Work on Himself in the Creative Process of Experiencing*). In order to justify such a leap, Stanislavsky devises a serious reason: the accident referred to above where Nazvanov, due to excessive agitation during a presentation, squeezed a glass ashtray and cut his hand. Analyzing what has happened and seeing it as the result of a student's overly-tensed body, Tortsov/Stanislavsky says to the young actors:

> I need to break the strict, systematic, theoretical sequence of our programme and tell you, earlier than intended, about one of the important elements in the actor's work – about the process of *muscle relaxation*.

---

[200]   Ramacharaka, *Hatha Yoga*, 182–88.
[201]   Kapsali, 146.

The real place for this question is where external technique, that is, work on the body, will be discussed. But the facts insistently state that it is more correct to turn to this question now, at the beginning of the programme, when it's a matter of internal technique, or, more accurately, of psycho-technique.[202]

It seems that not only the 'facts' (especially thought up by Stanislavsky himself) nudge Tortsov to such a sharp violation of the initially designed course structure, but also Stanislavsky's changing thoughts. It is reasonable to propose that the inclusion of the chapter about the relaxation of muscles into the book about internal psycho-technique reflected his developing understanding of acting as a holistic integral psycho-physiological-physical process. Indeed, according to the ideas of the early period of the System (and to the views of Ramacharaka, who affirmed that '*Raja Yoga*... holds that the internal world must be conquered before the outer world is attacked'),[203] Stanislavsky begins the training of the actor with internal technique. But there is no separation of the training of internal technique from the training of external technique in Stanislavsky's practice starting in the 1920s, and there could not be. According to the explanations of Tortsov, the relaxation of muscles is achieved in the first place by continual work of the *internal* 'observer or inspector'.[204] Further on, he proposes the mental isolation of a group of muscles (i.e. a task in the control of the body by the mind), exercises in movement, where only one group of muscles is involved (i.e. physical exercises) and the release from excess tension in the body through involving oneself in achieving a very challenging task (i.e. integral psychophysical 'training and drill'). One enumeration of this sequence of tasks is enough in order to understand that the chapter 'Relaxation of Muscles' rightfully belongs equally to both books – the one about internal as well as the one about external technique of the actor – and thereby reveals the unity

---

[202]   Stanislavskii, *Ss* 9, II (1989), 185.
[203]   Ramacharaka, *Raja Yoga*, 79.
[204]   Stanislavskii, *Ss* 9, II (1989), 188.

of the actor's work on himself. It also reveals the convention of dividing the book *An Actor's Work* into two volumes.

Furthermore, it is especially curious that Ramacharaka, likewise breaking the exposition of Yoga into two seemingly contrasting-in-content books (*Hatha Yoga* and *Raja Yoga*), cannot and does not want to follow the formal division of work on the mind and work on the body. In the Fourth Lesson of *Raja Yoga*, 'Mental Control', we read:

> It is well to accompany the above exercises with a comfortable and easy physical attitude, so as to prevent the distraction of the attention by the body. In order to do this one should assume an easy attitude, and then *relax every muscle*, and *take the tension from every nerve*, until a perfect sense of ease, comfort and relaxation is obtained [italics are mine].[205]

Thus, the importance of relaxation – within the practice of Yoga as well as in actor training – exposes the integral relationship between body and mind as well as the holistic nature of both approaches.[206]

Communication and Prana[207]

The concept of *prana* was one of Stanislavsky's most important borrowings from Yoga. This Sanskrit word (translated as 'wind', 'breath', 'life') in the philosophy of Yoga means the life force of a person, the soul. According to Yoga, the rays of the energy of life (*prana*) are subject to conscious control, and it is emission of *prana rays* that becomes for Stanislavsky the means of securing genuine communication for an actor.

---

[205]   Ramacharaka, *Raja Yoga*, 86.
[206]   Interestingly enough, Kapsali, who also draws attention to the above-mentioned parallels, considers that 'the importance of relaxation [...] forces both Atkinson and Stanislavski to *compromise* [italics are mine] "the strict, systematic, theoretical sequence" of their respective courses'. Kapsali, 146.
[207]   'Communication' (*obshchenie*) – a term of the System introduced by Stanislavsky in Chapter X of *An Actor's Work*. Hapgood (1936) translates it as 'communion'; Benedetti (2008) translates it as 'communication'.

Carnicke justly observes that for Stanislavsky *prana rays* became 'the vehicle for infecting others with the emotional content of the performance'.[208]

According to Ramacharaka's definition, familiar to Stanislavsky:

> Prana is the name by which we designate a universal principle, which principle is the essence of all motion, force or energy, whether manifested in gravitation, electricity, the revolution of the planets, and all forms of life, from the highest to the lowest. It may be called the soul of Force and Energy in all their forms, and that principle which, operating in a certain way, causes that form of activity which accompanies Life.
>
> This great principle is in all forms of matter, and yet it is not matter itself. It is in the air, but it is not the air, nor one of its chemical constituents. It is in the food we eat, and yet it is not the same as the nourishing substances in the food. It is in the water we drink, and yet it is not one or more of the chemical substances which combining make water. It is in the sunlight, but yet it is not the heat or the light rays. It is the 'energy' in all these things – the things acting merely as a carrier.[209]

According to Yoga principles, it is precisely *prana rays* that are emitted and received during spiritual or non-verbal communication.

We can only imagine how pleased Stanislavsky must have been to find parallels between the yogic tenets about *prana* and the ideas he had absorbed from the French psychologist Théodule Ribot, who provided the System not only with the concept of 'affective memory', but also with the terms 'immanation' and 'emanation', or 'emission of rays' and 'reception of rays', paramount for the description of the communicative process according to Stanislavsky. In their commentary to the manuscript of 1916–1920, *An Actor's Work on a Role (Woe from Wit)*, Kristi and Prokofev write that these terms were borrowed by Stanislavsky from Ribot's book *The Psychology of Attention*, excerpts from which are preserved in

[208] Carnicke, 178.
[209] Ramacharaka, *Hatha Yoga*, 152.

Stanislavsky's archive.[210] Despite the fact that Ribot does not employ the concept of *prana*, his idea of emanation is nothing else but a description, in different words, of the phenomenon of the exchange of energy. In the introduction to *The Psychology of Attention*, which Stanislavsky learned about in 1908, i.e. earlier than when he read *Hatha Yoga*, Ribot argues that the mechanism of the spiritual life of man

> consists of inner processes always replacing one another, and of the series of sensations, feelings, thoughts, and images, subject to either mutual association or mutual repulsion under the influence of well-known laws. Actually, this is not a chain or a series, as it is often expressed, but more like *emanation* [italics are mine] in different directions, permeating various layers.[211]

It should be mentioned that the idea of rays permeating the space around us concerned many representatives of Russian art at the beginning of the twentieth century. This is not odd because in 1897 Alexander Popov transmitted radio waves for the first time, and the ideas about the possibility of emanation and reception of invisible rays started to appear in everyday life. In 1913, the artist Mikhail Larionov (1881–1964) published the manifesto of a new movement in painting, 'Rayonism' (*Luchism* in Russian), the goal of which was 'to convey the fourth dimension', to catch, to depict on the canvas rays as the reflection of 'the inner essence of objects'.[212] Thus a technical discovery at the beginning of the twentieth century added a new dimension to the centuries-old yogic knowledge about the nature of man. Contemporary science has experimentally confirmed the existence of human bio-energy available for emanation. Consequently, basic concepts of the Stanislavsky

---

[210] Stanislavskii, *Ss* 8, IV (1957), 490.
[211] Théodule Ribot, *Psikhologiia vnimaniia* (Saint Petersburg: F. Pavlenkov, 1897), 5. In his book, Gippius offers a somewhat clearer translation of this paragraph: 'The mechanism of mental life consists of the incessant change of inner processes, of the range of sensations, feelings, ideas, and images which unify with each other and repulse each other, following certain laws... This is what we mean by radiation in different directions and different layers, a flexible aggregate, being incessantly formed, destroyed and formed again'. See S. V. Gippius, *Akterskii trening. Gimnastika chuvstv*, 292.
[212] M. F. Larionov, *Luchism* (Moscow: K. and K., 1913).

System – 'emission rays', 'receiving rays', 'emanation' – have ceased to be perceived as purely imaginary, and, as Gracheva observes, 'in the contemporary scientific context they no longer appear supernatural'.[213]

Let us look at examples of the use of the concept of *prana* in Stanislavsky. In the chapter 'Communication' of the first part of *An Actor's Work on Himself* Stanislavsky defines the types of communication – with an object, with oneself, with a fellow actor, with the audience – and ascribes monologues, spoken when fellow actors are absent from the stage, to the second form of communication, 'self-communication'. However, from his own experience Stanislavsky knows that an actor who lacks a fellow actor is most often incapable of creating in himself two 'communicating centres', and is incapable of maintaining 'scattered, unfocused attention', thus, as a consequence, he slides down into theatrically stylized declamation. The problem seems almost unsolvable.

'How to justify on stage something that I can hardly find justification for in real life?', Tortsov asks, as if preparing a striking stage denouement.[214] He continues:

> However, I *was taught* [italics are mine] how to solve this problem. The fact is that, besides the usual centre of our neuro-psychic life, the brain, I *was pointed to* [italics are mine] another centre located near the heart, where the solar plexus is. I tried to bring together for conversation both centres. It seemed that not only did they take shape in me, but they even started speaking. The centre in the brain felt to me like the representative of the conscious, and the centre at the solar plexus, as the representative of emotion. Thus, according to my sensations, it turned out that the mind was communicating with feeling.[215]

Who was this person who 'taught' the System's creator and 'pointed' him? It is easy to uncover Stanislavsky's deliberate failure to mention his 'Master Teacher'. He is, of course,

---

[213]   L. V. Gracheva, *Trening vnutrennei svobody. Aktualizatsiia tvorcheskogo potentsiala* (Saint Petersburg: Rech, 2005), 5.
[214]   Stanislavskii, *Ss* 9, II (1989), 323.
[215]   *Ibid*.

Ramacharaka. In *Hatha Yoga* Stanislavsky had a chance to read about the solar plexus as a 'great central storehouse of Prana'.[216]

It seems that he also did not miss Ramacharaka's assertion that

> The Yogi teachings go further than does Western Science, in one important feature of the Nervous System. We allude to what Western science terms the 'Solar Plexus', and which it considers as merely one of a series of certain matted nets of sympathetic nerves with their ganglia found in various parts of the body. Yogi science teaches that this Solar Plexus is really a most important part of the Nervous System, and that it is a form of brain, playing one of the principal parts in the human economy.[217]

Ramacharaka justly emphasizes that 'the name "Solar" is well bestowed on this "brain", as it radiates strength and energy to all parts of the body, even the upper brains depending largely upon it as a storehouse of Prana'.[218]

The knowledge Stanislavsky gained took on a different aspect in a peculiar way in the chapter 'Communication' of *An Actor's Work on Himself in the Creative Process of Experiencing*. According to Stanislavsky, the genuine exchange of energy among actors occurring during emission and reception of rays is perceived by the audience as a confirmation of the instantaneous *truth of experiencing*. Besides that, there is an exchange of energy rays between actors and audiences. As Tortsov explains:

> If we could see with the help of some sort of device the process of immanation and emanation, which the stage and the house exchange at the moment of the flash of inspiration, we would be surprised by the fact that our nerves manage to endure the pressure of the *current* [another synonym for the word prana used in 1936; italics are mine], which we, the actors, send out to the audience and receive back from a thousand living organisms sitting in the stalls![219]

[216] Ramacharaka, *Hatha Yoga*, 158.
[217] *Ibid.*, 157–58.
[218] *Ibid.*, 158.
[219] Stanislavskii, *Ss* 9, II (1989), 347.

In March, 1912, it was no longer Tortsov but Stanislavsky himself who wrote down that he performed the sixth performance of *A Provincial Lady* by Turgenev according to the System, and 'thanks to the communication with the solar plexus [I] felt well. And the acting went well.'[220]

Let us note, by the way, that Tortsov/Stanislavsky's dreams about 'a device' were destined to come true. At the end of the twentieth century the human bio-field was indeed measured with the help of instruments.[221] Just one example: Gracheva reports that at the Institute of Precision Mechanics and Optics

> a group of Saint Petersburg scientists led by K. G. Korotkov created an instrument named 'Corona TV', which allows one to record and to register the changes of the psychophysical states on the basis of the analysis of the space, colour and defects of luminescence around the human body, the so-called 'aura'.[222]

It is this instrument that helped the researchers of the Laboratory of Psychophysiology of Performing Arts of the Saint Petersburg State Theatre Arts Academy not only to measure certain parameters of bio-energy and 'radiation' around an actor in the process of creating, but also come to some interesting conclusions about the dynamics in the changes of the psychophysical characteristics of students in the process of study.[223]

Prana, according to Stanislavsky, is of crucial importance not only in the process of actors' communication on stage. All plasticity and its spirituality are connected with *prana*. As already mentioned above, Grigorii Kristi, in his commentary to the third volume of Stanislavsky's *Collected Works*, writes about replacing the word *prana* with the more 'scholarly' word *energy*. He thereby gives us a clue to the whole book.

---

[220] I. N. Vinogradskaia, *Zhizn' i tvorchestvo K. S. Stanislavskogo* (Moscow: MXAT, 2003), II, 332.

[221] 'Bio-field' is a modern way to describe an electro-magnetic field surrounding a human body. Compare this with 'aura' (a fine emanation in the form of a white or coloured luminescence around the body of a living being).

[222] Gracheva, *Akterskii trening*, 12.

[223] *Ibid.*, 10.

Reading *An Actor's Work on Himself*, we understand that when Tortsov says 'that at the base of movement we should place not the visible external, but the invisible internal movement of energy [...] This inner feeling of the energy moving through the body we call the feeling of movement [i.e. prana]',[224] it means that here and further on we encounter the yogic foundation of the System.

In the manuscript of the mid-1930s, 'The Programme of the Theatre School and the Notes on Actor Training', Stanislavsky drafts a section, whose contents were yet to be developed, in the following way: 'The feeling of movement (prana)'.[225] He points out: 'Actors should *feel* [italics by Stanislavsky] their movements, will, emotions, and thoughts so that their will forces them to perform this or that movement (prana), so that the movements are not senseless.'[226] Thus, whenever Stanislavsky speaks about the movement training of an actor, about developing in him the feeling of movement, he approaches this question from a position initially adopted from Yoga.

Using an example – drawn from Stanislavsky's rehearsal practice of the late period – where an actor's movement and even his very existence on stage were connected with *prana rays*, Galendeev writes:

> We know and understand poorly the ways long-term human predilections arise, their 'source is mysteriously hidden'. Indeed, why was Stanislavsky so partial to cantilena, the uninterrupted melodious line in sound, word, movement, action? We can suppose that this uninterrupted line was in his thinking that very channel through which the spiritual energy, prana, could pass without spilling or hesitation and freely pour out.[227]

Thus Yoga, 'having united' with Ribot's theory, joins the list of scientific sources for the System. At the same time we should deflect possible accusations of eclecticism in Stanislavsky's

---

[224] Stanislavskii, *Ss 8*, III (1955), 49.
[225] *Ibid.*, 420.
[226] *Ibid.*, 394.
[227] Galendeev, 105.

views; he does not draw into the embrace of the System all of
the scientific information available to him. Moreover, even the
word 'science' sometimes raises his suspicion. According to
Olga Radischeva's account, during the lectures in November
1919 for the Moscow Art Theatre actors,

> Stanislavsky explained that science will not help the art of
> experiencing. 'Science now reigns in art completely', he said,
> meaning 'all of those triangles which Meyerhold draws'. They,
> in his opinion, only hinder the nature of creation. Stanislavsky
> sought help from other areas of science: psychology, physiology,
> and the teaching of yogis.[228]

Of course, Stanislavsky was attracted to only one kind of
science – the science of humanology.[229] And the facts of any
scientific knowledge accessible to him were verified by his
own actor's experience.

Let us now move on to the tenets that attracted Stanislavsky's
interest in Ramacharaka's *Raja Yoga*, those which deal with
the sixth and seventh steps of yogi Patanjali.

Attention[230]

From *Raja Yoga* Stanislavsky drew specific ways of sharpen-
ing concentration of attention and one's power of observation.
The centuries-old yogic techniques of attention on many

[228] O. A. Radischeva, *Stanislavskii i Nemirovich-Danchenko: Istoriia teatral-nykh otnoshenii, 1917–1938*, 60.
[229] 'Humanology' is a neologism coined in Russian many years ago to describe the study of humans. My teacher Prof. Sulimov borrowed it from the First Studio member Smyshliaev. Following Stanislavsky himself he usually insisted that 'the art of directing is the art of *humanology*', thus underlining that theatre is first of all the *study* of humans, not entertainment, and directing is first of all connected with a deep analysis of the human soul, and only secondly with the staging of the production. This position obviously represents Stanislavsky's actor-centered approach to theatre.
[230] 'Attention' (*vnimanie*) – Stanislavsky talks about this element of the System in Chapter V of *An Actor's Work*, called in Russian 'Stage Attention'. Hapgood (1936) translates it as 'concentration of attention'; Benedetti (2008) translates it as 'attention'. Some translations have it as 'concentration'.

planes, the practical devices for developing focus, seemed well suited to be used for the development of an actor's psycho-technique. In their exercises on attention training, yogis taught how to overcome distractions. They taught one to control one's attention, not to allow absent-mindedness, which manifests itself both when thought constantly jumps from one object to another, and when a person who is totally focused on one thought or object does not notice anything else.

Stanislavsky includes yogic exercises in Chapter Five, 'Stage Attention', of *An Actor's Work on Himself in the Creative Process of Experiencing*. The unintentional coincidences between the texts start to look symbolic: it is Lesson Five of *Raja Yoga* that is titled 'The Cultivation of Attention'. Both Stanislavsky and Ramacharaka start with traditional yogic exercises, which include focusing on an object, and retaining in memory the details of its appearance and qualities after the object is removed from one's field of vision. Further, Stanislavsky develops these exercises, adjusting them to the needs of the stage, and introduces the concept he already worked out of 'the circle of attention', which is so necessary for an actor to achieve concentration and 'public solitude' in the presence of an audience. It was essential for Stanislavsky that an actor not think about himself nor about the impression he makes on the audience, but concentrates on his task and fellow actors. Excessive self-control is the source of many problems of an actor.

It is surprising, but Ramacharaka was also aware of this problem and wrote in his Lesson Five about an actor's work. He gives advice to anyone who has to work in front of an audience: 'The actor, or preacher, or orator, or writer, must lose sight of himself to get the best results. Keep the Attention fixed on the thing before you, and let the self take care of itself.'[231]

---

[231] Ramacharaka, *Raja Yoga,* 111–12.

In Stanislavsky's Chapter Five, speaking about the circles of attention and public solitude, Tortsov retells 'a Hindu *fairy-tale*' (at this point we picture Stanislavsky smiling when this word-mask, serving as a disguise for one of the yogic sutras, comes into his head):

> The maharaja was choosing a minister. He will choose the one who can walk along the top of the wall around the city and carry a big jar filled to the brim with milk without spilling a drop. Many tried, but during their walk people called to them, frightened them and distracted them, so they spilled the milk.
>
> 'These are not ministers', maharaja said.
>
> But, here came a man. Neither shouts, nor frights, nor tricks could distract him from the overfilled jar.
>
> 'Shoot!' shouted the maharaja.
>
> They shot, but it did not help.
>
> 'Now this is a minister!' the maharaja said.
>
> 'Did you hear shouts?' he asked the man.
>
> 'No!'
>
> 'Did you see how they were trying to frighten you?'
>
> 'No. I was watching the milk.'
>
> 'Did you hear the shots?'
>
> 'No, Your Majesty! I was watching the milk.'
>
> Tortsov finished this story: this is what it means to be in the circle! This is what true attention is, and not in the dark, but in the light![232]

What is this yogic example about, if not about *the public solitude in the circle of attention*?

It is worth noting a similar episode from Yogananda's book where a young man, having achieved the same feeling of being 'in the circle' amidst the hustle and bustle of Calcutta finds himself suddenly enveloped in 'a transforming silence' when 'pedestrians as well as the passing trolley cars, automobiles, bullock carts, and iron-heeled hackney carriages were all in noiseless transit'.[233]

---

[232] Stanislavskii, *Ss* 9, II (1989), 164.
[233] Paramahansa Yogananda, *Autobiography of a Yogi* (Los Angeles: Self-Realization Fellowship, 1993), 94–95. Quoted in Carnicke, 178.

Visualizations (Mental images)[234]

This important element of the System is connected with the meditative techniques of Yoga. Stanislavsky's ideas about the necessity of 'inner visions', about the creation of a 'filmstrip of visions', about the significance of artistic 'dreams', are inseparable from another element of the creative sense of self: 'imagination', which is analyzed in Chapter Four of *An Actor's Work on Himself in the Creative Process of Experiencing.*

Out of many examples from this chapter let us pay attention to the task given to the students: to imagine oneself being a tree. Tortsov tries to have the students make the vision concrete, specifying the kind of tree, its height, colour, and size of its leaves, making the students imagine insects and birds in the branches of the tree, feel the roots going deep into the soil and the branches reaching to the clear sky. Further, sensory feelings are added which are connected to the weather, the surrounding woods, the height of the hill on top of which an ancient oak stands alone, the time of year, and even the time in history. And so the student, merging in his imagination with a powerful oak, *sees* himself surrounded by knights, *sees* a noisy celebration, an enemy's attack, and is seriously *frightened* by the enemy's attempt to cut him down and burn him!

Itemizing the visions, Stanislavsky/Tortsov lures the students' imagination into the territory beyond the limits of their personal experience, into the world unknown to them which they would not be able to get to know otherwise than through their imagination and visions.[235]

The choice of the subject for this focused dream, for this meditation, is probably connected with the Hindu ideas

---

[234] 'Visualizations' (*videniia*) – a term of the System introduced by Stanislavsky in the chapter 'Imagination' of *An Actor's Work*. Hapgood (1936) translates it as 'images'; Benedetti (2008) translates it as 'mental images'. In some translations, you might find 'visualizations' (Carnicke) and 'visions'.

[235] Stanislavskii, *Ss* 9, II (1989), 133–36.

about the interpenetration between our being and everything
that surrounds it. According to Tagore:

> In the West the prevalent feeling is that nature belongs
> exclusively to inanimate things and to beasts, that there is a
> sudden unaccountable break where human-nature begins.
> Proceeding from such an approach, everything that is lower on
> the scale of development is merely wild nature, and whatever
> has the stamp of perfection on it, intellectual or moral, is
> connected with man. It is like ascribing the bud and the blossom
> to different categories, and linking their grace with two different
> and antithetical principles. But the Indian mind never has any
> hesitation in acknowledging its kinship with nature, its unbroken
> relation with all.[236]

Today, when we habitually conduct exercises in which
the students impersonate animals, plants, objects and even
stones,[237] we sometimes do not even think how revolutionary
was this extension of the thematic territory of actor training,
undertaken by Stanislavsky in the First Studio under the
influence of the Eastern world-outlook.

More than that, Stanislavsky's ideas about thinking by
means of inner visions and about the existence of a chain
of such visions (which he names a 'filmstrip of visions', and
which pave the way to the through-line of an actor's existence)
anticipated the ideas of modern neurobiology. A leading
representative of this field of science of the late twentieth
century, Antonio Damasio, discussing how 'the brain gives
birth to inner pictures which we name images of objects',
writes:

> Quite candidly, this first problem of consciousness is the problem
> of how we get a 'movie-in-the-brain', provided we realize that in

---

[236] Rabindranath Tagore, *Sādhanā* (New York: Doubleday, 2004), 4.
[237] One of the exercises of the first-year actor training at the Saint Petersburg
Theatre Arts Academy is called 'Stones'. It enables students – who are forced to
be immobile due to the nature of the objects they are exploring and presenting
– to understand clearly the richness of the inner life of their characters (stones
on a hill that are experiencing the conditions of nature and the wild life around)
even when it is not expressed outwardly. See V. M. Filshtinskii, *Otkrytaia
pedagogika* (Saint Petersburg: Baltiiskie Sezoni, 2006), 38–42.

this rough metaphor the movie has as many sensory tracks as our nervous system has sensory portals – sight, sound, taste, and olfaction, touch, inner senses, and so on.[238]

Carnicke broadens Damasio's 'so on': 'Stanislavsky would find emotional memory implicit in this list of senses as well.'[239]

Let us also point out another possible source – one quite distant from Yoga! – of Stanislavsky's ideas about visions: the views of the Roman orator of the first century CE Marcus Fabius Quintilianus, who, like Aristotle, supposed that the process of thinking happens through a sequence of inner images.[240]

This example underlines, once and for all, that, although this book examines the rapport between the elements of the System and Yoga, the elaboration of almost every element of the System could have been inspired by many sources. The main source, which we are not discussing here, but which we should not forget for a moment, is Stanislavsky's own experience as an actor, one of the greatest of the twentieth century, enhanced by his unique talent as a researcher and teacher.

Superconscious

Besides the aforementioned elements – relaxation of muscles, communication, attention, visualizations/mental images – familiarization with the theory and practice of Yoga enriched the System with elements that had not been present in it before. From *Raja Yoga* Stanislavsky drew the idea of the connection between the creative state and the unconscious state, borrowing the idea of the superconscious as a source of creative intuition and transcendental knowledge. This

---

[238] Antonio Damasio, *The Feeling of What Happens: Body and Emotion in the Making of Consciousness* (New York: Penguin, 1999), 9. As cited in Carnicke, 178.

[239] Carnicke, 178.

[240] Joseph Roach, *The Player's Passion* (Newark: University of Delaware Press, 1985), 24–25.

idea permeates all of Stanislavsky's pursuits starting from the mid-1910s. The slogan 'the unconscious through the conscious', proclaimed at the first rehearsal of *The Village of Stepanchikovo* by Dostoyevsky (1916), was henceforth repeated by the creator of the System multiple times as an incantation. As we have already seen, at the end of his life, in the introduction to the first volume of *An Actor's Work on Himself* (1938), Stanislavsky points to the key meaning of Chapter Sixteen of the book which, for him, contains 'the essence of creativity and of the whole System'. The title of this chapter is 'The Subconscious in the Sense of Self of an Actor on Stage'.

According to the conceptions of yogis, the unconscious life of man is divided into two components: the subconscious that exists in every man and the superconscious that goes beyond the individual, a sort of higher consciousness, the area of the transcendental. In Stanislavsky's opinion, art makes contact with this Highest component, half-opens it, and that is why it can speak across cultures, centuries and individual differences. All the emotional and, dare we say, religious pathos of Stanislavsky concerning 'the mysteries of life-giving nature', all the understanding of theatre is connected with the discovery of this wondrous phenomenon of the human psyche.

At the same time the role of the superconscious, according to Stanislavsky, in the array of elements comprising the creative sense of self is so significant that many theatre researchers who are not familiar with the connections between the Stanislavsky System and yogic teaching are sure that it was Stanislavsky who introduced this concept and the very term the 'superconscious' to the psychology and the studies of an actor's creativity. We come across such statements in the works by Ned Manderino[241] and John Sullivan. The latter writes: 'The term "superconscious", which appears

---

[241] Ned Manderino, *Stanislavski's Fourth Level: A Superconscious Approach to Acting* (Los Angeles: Manderino Books, 2001), 4.

in Stanislavsky's writing, is a genuine original. It does not appear in any well-established system of psychology.'[242]

However, Stanislavsky himself, speaking about this subject which was very important for him, already in the manuscript of the late 1910s, *An Actor's Work on a Role (Woe from Wit)*, immediately reveals the origins of his views and takes yogis as his allies. Thus, arguing in the chapter 'The Superconscious' that 'the only approach to the unconscious is through the conscious' and that 'the only approach to the superconscious, the unreal, is through the real, through the ultra-natural, i.e. through organic nature',[243] Stanislavsky reveals the source of his understanding of the matter:

> The Hindu yogis, achieving miracles in the areas of sub- and superconscious, give much practical advice in this area. They also approach the unconscious through conscious preparative devices, from the material to the spiritual, from the real to the unreal, from naturalism to the abstract. And we, artists, should do the same.[244]

Stanislavsky, however, never gives strict definitions of what the superconscious and the subconscious are. The reason might be that every artist, at least once in his life, has experienced the great power of inspiration when the subconscious itself comes into its own. One, who has never experienced this, will not grasp it, no matter what explanation of it is made.

In the discussion about this element of 'our miraculous nature', Stanislavsky is closer to the approach that employs images. Thus, the final chapter of the American edition of *An Actor's Work on Himself – An Actor Prepares* (1936), titled 'On the Threshold of the Subconscious' (in the Russian version, 'The Subconscious in the Sense of Self of an Actor on Stage') contains a number of Tortsov's remarks, which were removed from the Russian edition either by the censors or by Stanislavsky himself because of their obvious spiritual tone. When Nazvanov is

[242] John Sullivan, 'Stanislavski and Freud' in *Stanislavski and America*, ed. by Erika Munk (New York: Hill and Wang, 1966), 104.
[243] Stanislavskii, *Ss* 8, IV (1957), 156.
[244] *Ibid.*, 157.

· 96 ·

working on the etude 'Burning Money' and immerses himself more deeply in the given circumstances, he, in Tortsov's words, finds himself on the shore of 'the ocean of the subconscious'. Tortsov employs metaphors to evaluate the work of his student, speaking about these tidal waves. When Nazvanov, absorbed in his thoughts, mechanically twists a bit of string around his finger, Tortsov says that the student is 'on the threshold'; when a chance glance at the clock sharply activates the rhythm of the performer's life, Tortsov speaks about 'the big wave'; when the inner monologue of Nazvanov, rushing about in search of an exit from the situation taking shape, bursts outside with separate words, Tortsov comments that 'the water is up to his waist now'. And when Nazvanov unexpectedly immerses himself in concentrated immobility, Tortsov whispers to the other students: 'Now he is in the very depth of the ocean of the subconscious.'[245] As Carnicke points out,

> In the Western context, this image easily calls to mind Freud's analysis of religiosity as an 'oceanic feeling', and, in fact, the connection to religious sentiment is apt. While Stanislavsky would reject a dark, Freudian view of the subconscious, he would embrace this spiritual association. Tolstoyan 'experiencing' as the desired state of the actor in performance shares much with Eastern spirituality; recall Yogananda's description of his meditative moment as 'oceanic joy'. [...] The actor, like the yogi, engulfed by the creative state of mind, undergoes something akin, when mind, body, and soul unite in communion, not only with each other, but also with others on stage and those present in the audience.[246]

For a long period of time Stanislavsky's commentators have tried to suggest that the terms 'superconscious' and 'subconscious' are synonyms. For example, the notes to the fourth volume of the *Collected Works* published in 1957 inform us that 'superconscious'

> is a term uncritically borrowed by Stanislavsky from idealistic philosophy and psychology. At the end of the 1920s Stanislavsky

---

[245] Stanislavski, Constantin, *An Actor Prepares*, trans. by Elizabeth Reynolds Hapgood (New York: Theatre Arts Books, 1936), 274–75.
[246] Carnicke, 167.

rejected the term 'superconscious' and replaced it with the term 'subconscious', which more precisely expresses his views of the nature of the actor's creativity and corresponds with modern scientific terminology.[247]

However, Smeliansky is right, saying that today 'not only theatre scholars, but psychologists, too, are trying to interpret in a scientific way some of Stanislavsky's practical observations, in particular his persistent division of the concepts of "the subconscious" and "the superconscious" of an actor'.[248] Smeliansky cites the point of view of Pavel Simonov, who thinks that 'Stanislavsky in this case does not simply use synonyms, but also comes across an extraordinarily deep and essential difference between the two mechanisms involved in the creative act.'[249] According to this scholar, author of the landmark work *K. S. Stanislavsky's Method and the Physiology of Emotion* (1962), the superconscious is a special kind of extramental psychic. If the subconscious governs, so to speak, exclusively individual adjustments of the organism, automatic skills, shades of emotions and their outward expression, then, 'the superconscious deals with those areas of reality whose pragmatic value is doubtful, unclear'.[250]

Thus, Smeliansky concludes that the superconscious of an actor is

> the area of discoveries, inventions, news. The superconscious discovers the unknown, the subconscious comes up with a cliché. In the superconscious the craziest creative projects are formed, the most unexpected artistic hypotheses, which to a great extent counterbalance the conservatism of the conscious which guards us from everything accidental, suspicious, not approved by practice'.[251]

---

[247] Stanislavskii, *Ss* 8, IV (1957), 495.
[248] Smeliansky in Stanislavskii, *Ss* 9, II (1989), 26.
[249] *Ibid.*
[250] P. V. Simonov, 'Kategoriia soznaniia, podsoznaniia i sverkhsoznaniia v tvorcheskoi sisteme K. S. Stanislavskogo', *Bessoznatelnoe. Priroda. Funktsii. Metody Issledovaniia*, II (Tbilisi: Metsniereba, 1978). Cited in Smeliansky in Stanislavskii, *Ss* 9, II (1989), 26.
[251] Smeliansky in Stanislavskii, *Ss* 9, II (1989), 26–27.

It is worth mentioning that the question of the correlation between the conscious and the unconscious is central for Yoga teaching too. For example Swami Vivekananda,[252] whose charismatic appearance at the World's Parliament of Religions in Chicago in 1893 triggered American enthusiasm for Yoga, interpreted Yoga (also trying to bring it closer to Western mentality) as 'the method of changing the interrelations between consciousness (*vritti*) and psychic phenomena pertaining to the sphere of the unconscious (*sanskari vasana*)'.[253] Perhaps because of this Stanislavsky's dialogue with Yoga turned out to be so fruitful.

However, it was not only Yoga teaching that brought Stanislavsky to an understanding of the psychic life of man and the balance between his conscious and unconscious life. Equal with Yoga as the source of Stanislavsky's ideas about the unconscious could be the works of the German philosopher Eduard von Hartmann (1842–1906), whose book *The Philosophy of the Unconscious* (1869) was remarkably popular in Russia for many years. According to Hartmann, there are three levels of the unconscious:

1. the absolute unconscious which constitutes the substance of the universe and is the source of other forms of the unconscious;

2. the physiological unconscious, which is at work in the origin, development, and evolution of living beings, including man;

3. the relative or psychological unconscious, which lies at the source of our conscious mental life.[254]

---

[252] Swami Vivekananda (1863–1902) was a Hindu philosopher and social activist, a pupil of Ramakrishna, a key figure in the introduction of Vedanta and Yoga philosophies to the Western world, and the founder of the Ramakrishna Mission. At the time of the four-year tour of 1893–1897, he founded the Vedanta Centres in New York and London.

[253] V. S. Kostiuchenko, *Vivekananda* (Moscow: Misl, 1977), 124.

[254] See Henri Ellenberger, *The Discovery of the Unconscious* (New York: Basic Books, 1970), 210. Also cited in Whyman, 89.

It is not hard to draw parallels: Stanislavsky's superconscious corresponds to Hartmann's absolute unconscious;
Stanislavsky's unconscious to Hartmann's physiological unconscious; and subconscious to the psychological unconscious. Although some scholars claim that Stanislavsky took
the term 'superconscious' exclusively from Yoga,[255] others are
confident that he was also influenced by a similar structuring
of the unconscious that existed in European thought of
Stanislavsky's day.[256] It must not be ruled out that such
'mixing' from different sources was possible for Stanislavsky
because, creating Ramacharaka's books, Atkinson himself
freely mixed yogic traditions with more contemporary
theories. The resulting merging of Western and Eastern
views of the phenomenon of the unconscious turned out to
be quite fruitful. In Stanislavsky's private library there are
excerpts from Sergei Sukhanov's article of 1915 entitled 'The
Subconscious and Its Pathology' (this selection was prepared
for Stanislavsky by the Moscow Art Theatre actor Vladimir
Gaidarov).[257] Sukhanov's article discusses the interrelations
between the conscious 'I' and the subconscious in the context
of information gained from the study of pathologic conditions.
It is curious that the image of 'the sack of the subconscious',
which, as we already know, was borrowed by Stanislavsky
from *Hatha Yoga*, is encountered here as well.

To summarize, Stanislavsky drew from many sources.
Examining the phenomenon of memory, he, 'like Von Hartmann,
[…] sees memory as a storehouse of the unconscious, and like
Sechenov[258] sees memory as receiving traces or impressions of
stimuli from the outside world, which we receive through the

---

[255]   See, for example, Carnicke, 179–80.
[256]   For details see Whyman, 89–90, where the following parallels of
Hartmann's, Sechenov's, and Sukhanov's works with Stanislavsky's ideas are
discussed.
[257]   S. L. Sukhanov, 'Podsoznanie i ego patologiia', *Voprosy filosofii i psikhologii*,
26 (128) (1915), 362–77.
[258]   Ivan Sechenov (1829–1905), a Russian physiologist whose works laid the
foundations for the study of reflexes and neuroscience.

sense organs in our nervous system'.[259] This is, for instance, what Stanislavsky wrote about his childhood encounter with opera when he found 'the music boring': 'The power of the impressions itself was huge, not realized then, but perceived organically and unconsciously, *not only spiritually, but physically as well* [italics are mine]. I understood and appreciated these impressions only afterwards, based on memories.'[260]

In any event, following the connections between the System, and Yoga, and German philosophy of the nineteenth century, we can restore Stanislavsky's initial thought. As Simonov writes:

> having insightfully grasped the infeasibility of gathering under the term 'subconscious' everything that is hard to realize – from the activities of the inner organs to creative insights – the great and deep thinker K. S. Stanislavsky felt a real need for some other concept, which would signify only the highest and most complex mechanisms of creation. He called the last category of the unrealizable processes the 'superconscious'.[261]

Stanislavsky regards the subconscious as a way to the superconscious:

> in order to establish communication with his superconscious, an actor [as well as a yogi] should be able 'to take certain clusters of thoughts with the purpose of throwing them into his sack of the subconscious'. The food for the superconscious, the material for creation is contained in these 'certain clusters of thoughts.[262]

This example from Yoga is found both in the manuscript *An Actor's Work on a Role* (*Woe from Wit*) and in the rehearsals of Dostoyevsky's work.[263]

A large section from *An Actor's Work on a Role* – quoted in full below – gives an idea of the practical use of the ideas about

[259] Whyman, 89. See also I. M. Sechenov, *Reflexes of the Brain* (Cambridge: Massachusetts, 1965), 67–68.
[260] Stanislavskii, *Ss* 9, I (1988), 70.
[261] P. V. Simonov, 'Soznanie, podsoznanie, sverkhsoznanie', *Nauka i zhizn*, 12 (1975), 46.
[262] Stanislavskii, *Ss* 9, IV (1991), 144.
[263] Notes from rehearsals of *The Village of Stepanchikovo*, 12 January 1915, in *Stanislavskii repetiruet*, 73–74.

the existence of the unconscious. Of course, Stanislavsky was particularly interested in the mechanisms of control of the unconscious activities of the mind which does definite work of *thinking* and *imagination*, resulting in the birth of ideas and artistic images.

Stanislavsky wrote:

> The practical advice we are given by Hindu yogis regarding the superconscious sphere is in the following: take a certain cluster of thoughts, they say, and throw it into your sack of the subconscious; I do not have time to deal with this, therefore you (i.e. the subconscious) should deal with it. Then go to sleep, and when you wake up, ask: is it ready? – Not yet.
>
> Again, take the cluster of thoughts and throw it into the sack of the subconscious, etc. Then go for a walk and, coming back, ask: is it ready? – No. And so on and so on. In the end, the subconscious will say: ready, and will give back what it has been ordered to do [this is a retelling of Ramacharaka's thoughts[264]].
>
> How often we, going to bed or for a stroll, try in vain to remember a forgotten melody, or a thought, or a name, or an address, and tell ourselves: 'Sleep on it.' Indeed, waking up in the morning we seem to regain our sight and feel surprised at what happened overnight. Hence the saying – every thought has to spend the night in one's head. The work of our subconscious and superconscious does not stop at night (when our body and our whole nature rest) nor during the day amidst the hustle and bustle of everyday life, when both thought and feeling are distracted by other things. However, we do not see and do not know anything

---

[264] Ramacharaka wrote in *Raja Yoga*: 'The Yogi takes the student when the latter is much bothered by a consideration of some knotty and perplexing philosophical subject. He bids the student relax every muscle – take the tension from every nerve – throw aside all mental strain, and then wait a few moments. Then the student is instructed to grasp the subject which he has had before his mind, firmly and fixedly before his mental vision, by means of concentration. Then he is instructed to pass it on to the sub-conscious mentality by an effort of the Will, which effort is aided by forming a mental picture of the subject as a material substance, or *bundle of thought*, which is being bodily lifted up and dropped down a mental hatch-way, or trap-door, in which it sinks from sight. The student is then instructed to say to the sub-conscious mentality: "I wish this subject thoroughly analyzed, arranged, classified (and whatever else is desired) and then the results handed back to me. Attend to this."' (Ramacharaka, *Raja Yoga*, 229–30)

about this work, as it is outside our consciousness. [Modern psychology confirms that we may not be aware of a certain part of our mental activity, but this does not mean that it stops.]

Thus, in order to establish communication with one's superconscious, an actor has to be able 'to take certain clusters of thoughts with the purpose of throwing them into his sack of the subconscious'. The food for the superconscious, the material for creation is contained in these 'certain clusters of thoughts'.

What are these clusters of thoughts and where can we obtain them? They are in our knowledge, information, experience, memories, i.e. in the material preserved in our intellectual, affective, visual, auditory, muscle and other memories. That is why it is so important for an actor to replenish constantly these used-up materials, so that the storeroom is never left without a supply. [One can say without exaggeration that the fundamental tenets of the System, the yogis' superconscious and Ribot's affective memory, meet in these lines.]

That is why an actor must constantly replenish the store of his memory, [he must] study, read, observe, travel, be informed about modern social, religious, political and other life. From this material the clusters of thoughts come into being, which are then thrown into the unconscious sack in order to be processed by the superconscious. Providing the superconscious with work, one should not hurry it; one has to be able to be patient. Otherwise, as yogis say, what will happen is the same that happens to a silly child who, having thrown a seed into the soil, roots it out every half an hour in order to see whether it has taken root. [The example with a child is also a retelling of a fragment from Ramacharaka's *Raja Yoga*.[265]][266]

In his own experience, the actor Stanislavsky never once went through what the teacher Tortsov writes about. He knew well that at times it is worth giving up on a consciously supplied creative task which is not amenable to solution, and letting the answers arise by themselves. Examples of such

[265] Ramacharaka wrote in *Raja Yoga*: 'Do not make the mistake of yielding to the impatience of the beginner, and keep on repeatedly bringing up the matter to see what is being done. Give it time to have the work done on it. Do not be like the boy who planted seeds, and who each day would pull them up to see whether they had sprouted, and how much.' (Ramacharaka, *Raja Yoga*, 238)
[266] Stanislavskii, *Ss* 8, IV (1957), 158–59.

fruitful flashes of the subconscious are, first, the story of Stanislavsky's creation of the 'happy role' of Dr Stockmann in Ibsen's *Enemy of the People*. (Stanislavsky wrote, 'Life itself worried, in a timely fashion, about how to fulfil all the preparatory creative work and to store the necessary spiritual material'[267] and that is why 'the requirements and habits [of the character] appeared instinctively, unconsciously'.[268]) Second, a more particular episode is from Chapter Eight of *An Actor's Work on Himself in the Creative Process of Embodiment*, where Nazvanov unexpectedly senses the character named 'faultfinder' as a result of accidentally spoiled makeup.[269] ('I glanced in passing in the mirror and did not recognize myself […] a new regeneration had already been accomplished in me'; moreover, this formation of the character took place as if by itself: 'I myself was astonished…'[270]) Actually, the literature about theatre is full of stories about such creative epiphanies.

Thus, Stanislavsky's ideas about the subconscious are drawn from a series of sources, the priority of which can be evaluated differently. Carnicke and White see the basic source of influence on the author of the System to be precisely Yoga. Whyman considers that his ideas of the subconscious are rooted in European mid-nineteenth-century philosophy with an admixture of ideas from Sechenov and Ribot, and 'confirmed by his [Stanislavsky] reading on Yoga'.[271] Kapsali correctly emphasizes that it is a question of Modern Yoga and therefore she gives primacy to metaphysical thought:

> Taking into account the sources of Stanislavski's encounter with Yoga, the milieu in which these sources have been developed, as well as Stanislavski's interest in and influence by other systems of thought, it would be more accurate to support that what underlies the System and gives it its 'spiritual' character, is its

[267] Stanislavskii, *Ss* 9, I (1988), 319–20.
[268] *Ibid.*, 320–21.
[269] Stanislavskii, *Ss* 9, III (1990), 235–39.
[270] *Ibid.*, 235.
[271] Whyman, 91.

grounding – through Yoga – in nineteenth-century metaphysical thought.[272]

Despite the importance of the discussion about the correlation of various sources of scientific knowledge influencing Stanislavsky, it seems that Stanislavsky himself would have proved to be indifferent to the results of this debate. He would have been inclined to accentuate what the writings of Ramacharaka, Hartmann, Sukhanov, and Ribot had *in common*. Each of them in his own way described the mechanisms of the onset of inspiration owing to the preliminary work of the subconscious, and Stanislavsky skilfully separated out that which accorded with his practical experience. After all, in the process of accumulating new knowledge and using it in the actor's profession, he trusted in the first place his own internal tuning fork: 'to understand means to feel'. It is not for nothing, having described with humour in *An Actor's Work* the speechless communication of quarrelling lovers whom he had observed while paying a visit to relatives, and having caught the essence of the process that took place before his eyes (communication occurs through emission of rays and reception of rays), Stanislavsky steps away from further analysis: 'Let the people of science explain to us the nature of this invisible process, I can speak only about how I personally experience it in myself and how I make use of these sensations for my art.'[273]

That is why Stanislavsky, though without proposing a strict definition of the subconscious or the theory of its mechanism (as Vsevolod Meyerhold said, 'in art it is more important not to know, but to guess'),[274] actively includes the concepts of the unconscious, subconscious, and superconscious in the practical work of an actor. For him it is a mystery, governed by nature and indirectly accessible through the conscious

---

[272] Kapsali, 145–46.
[273] Stanislavskii, *Ss* 9, II (1989), 340.
[274] V. E. Meyerhold, *Stati, pisma, rechi, besedy*, 2 vols (Moscow: Iskusstvo, 1968), II, 113.

psycho-technique of an actor. Tortsov/Stanislavsky counsels his actors: 'We will leave all the subconscious to nature the enchantress, and will turn ourselves to that which is accessible to us, namely to the conscious approaches to creative work and to conscious devices of the psycho-technique.'[275]

'I am'[276]

In *An Actor's Work on a Role (Woe from Wit)*, referring to the authority of European scientists,[277] Stanislavsky identifies what for him is the most important aspect drawn from Yoga and which deeply coincides with his personal actor's experience: 'The superconscious elevates the human soul more than anything else and therefore should be most valued and guarded in our art.'[278]

Here, perhaps, is the main intersection of the Stanislavsky System and Yoga. For Yoga the superconscious is a sacred state through which an aspiring candidate in the end reaches the eighth and last limb of Patanjali Yoga, called *samadhi*. As Andrew White points out,

> multiple levels of samadhi exist; but the highest state of meditation is that in which the aspirant is completely absorbed by the object of meditation. For the Yogi, the object of meditation is God. For Stanislavsky, the object of meditation is the role.[279]

In order to convey this transcendental state of unity with the role, Stanislavsky introduces the concept 'I am'

---

[275] Stanislavskii, *Ss* 9, II (1989), 61.

[276] 'I am' (*ya esm*) – a term of the System introduced by Stanislavsky in the Chapter 'Imagination' of *An Actor's Work*. Hapgood (1936) avoids using and translating this phrase; Benedetti (2008) translates it as 'I am being'. More widespread translation is 'I am' (Carnicke, Whyman).

[277] Stanislavsky wrote, 'Professor Elmar Götz says, "At least ninety-nine percent of our mental life is subconscious." Maudsley establishes that "the conscious does not have even a tenth of those functions which are normally ascribed to it", Stanislavskii, *Ss* 9, IV (1991), 140.

[278] *Ibid.*, 140.

[279] White, 87.

(*ya esm*). In a sense, Stanislavsky's 'I am' is a synonym for the creative state of an actor in the process of true experiencing. Ironically, in contemporary Russian editions of Ramacharaka's *Raja Yoga* the concept 'I am', fundamental for him, is translated into Russian as *ya esm*. It turns out that now the language of Stanislavsky, known today to everyone if only through hearsay, helps one to assimilate the texts of Hindu wisdom.

This is how Ramacharaka introduces the division of the inner essence of man:

> The Yogi Masters teach that there are two degrees of this awakening consciousness of the Real Self. The first, which they call "the Consciousness of the 'I'", is the full consciousness of *real* existence that comes to the Candidate, and which causes him to *know* that he is a real entity having a life not depending upon the body – life that will go on in spite of the destruction of the body – real life, in fact. The second degree, which they call 'the Consciousness of the "I AM"', is the consciousness of one's identity with the Universal Life, and his relationship to, and 'intouchness' with all life, expressed and unexpressed.[280]

Here it seems that Stanislavsky finds a partial answer to the question that bothered him as early as 1906 when he realized the impossibility for an actor to separate the means of expression from the reality of his physical body. Yogis describe the inspired state of the conscious, when a student begins to see clearly the truth that the conscious not only exists separately from the material body, but will outlive it. Just as for Ramacharaka in the state of 'I am' there occurs a spiritual unity of the student with the universal energy of life, so for Stanislavsky in the state of 'I am' the unity of an actor with his role occurs, and in this state the feeling of awkwardness and concerns about his physical body go away. When an actor finds himself in the state of 'I am', 'the psychic and physical apparatus of an actor works on stage normally, according to

---

[280]   Ramacharaka, *Raja Yoga*, p. VI.

all the laws of human nature, exactly as in life, in spite of the abnormal conditions of public creativity'.[281]

It seems Stanislavsky makes the voice of Tortsov as Master Teacher become solemn when he answers the questions of his students aspiring to initiation, and he leads them along the path where, ascending the steps, they 'should find a small, genuine, human, life truth, giving rise to faith, creating the state 'I am':

'And what will happen then?'

'It will happen that you will experience vertigo caused by several moments of *the unexpected and complete merging of the life of the character you portray with your own life on stage*. It will happen that you will sense the particles of yourself in the role and the role – in yourself.'

'And then?'

'And then – what I have already told you: truth, faith, 'I am' will place you in the power of organic nature with its subconscious [italics are mine].'[282]

Here Stanislavsky's 'I am', in which 'the complete merging' of an actor and a role occurs, has something in common with the yogic *samadhi*, where the complete merging of a candidate with the divine takes place. Thus, in the single term of the System (*ya esm* – 'I am'), which comes from Church Slavonic, we can hear overtones of the sacred sound of yogic meditation, *om*.[283]

[281] Stanislavskii, *Ss* 9, II (1989), 439.

[282] *Ibid.*, 441.

[283] 'Om' (*aum*) is a sacred syllable in Hinduism that is considered to be the greatest of all the mantras, or sacred formulas. The syllable *om* is composed of the three sounds *a–u–m* (in Sanskrit, the vowels *a* and *u* coalesce to become *o*), which represent several important triads: the three worlds of earth, atmosphere, and heaven; thought, speech, and action; the three qualities of matter (goodness, passion, and darkness); etc. Thus, *om* mystically embodies the essence of the entire universe.

Conclusion

To summarize. If we compare the list of elements in the Stanislavsky System in which a yogic 'flavour' is present with the list of contents of *An Actor's Work on Himself in the Creative Process of Experiencing*, we find that we have listed about one third of the elements discussed in this book. This is quite a lot.

Creating – for the first time in the history of theatrical art – a system for an actor's creative work based on the laws of living nature and not on the aesthetic postulates of theatre of a specific period, Stanislavsky drew information from the body of knowledge accumulated by mankind up to that moment. The range of knowledge analyzed by him is impressive – from the lessons of Mikhail Shchepkin[284] and the realistic traditions of Russian theatre to the practice of Hatha Yoga and Raja Yoga, from the works of the Roman rhetorician Quintilianus to the psychological research of Théodule Ribot and treatises of classical German philosophy.

When Stanislavsky came across similar ideas in various sources, he saw one more confirmation of the precision of his pursuits. The same ideas circulated at the end of the nineteenth and the beginning of the twentieth centuries in science, philosophy, and art. Let us remember the characteristic message, cited above, of yogi Ramacharaka to Western science with an appeal to realize the significance of the solar plexus. Let us note that Ramacharaka himself was open to collaboration. Not only did he quote Ribot in *Raja Yoga*, but also argued that 'The Theory of the East, wedded to the practice of the West, will create worthy offspring.'[285] Probably that is why borrowing ideas from both Ribot and Yoga occurred so naturally for Stanislavsky, and he did not contrast Yoga with science. Moreover, they were brilliantly joined in Stanislavsky's theory and practice. Stanislavsky himself was well aware of this continuum: 'Everything I say

---

[284] Michael Shchepkin (1788–1863) was the most famous Russian actor of the nineteenth century known for many roles in the Maly Theatre.
[285] Ramacharaka, *Hatha Yoga*, 103.

is taken from psychology and physiology and confirmed by Yoga.' Thus, the System of the Russian theatre reformer was forged in the crucible of ideas from the French philosopher Ribot and the American yogi.

The contribution of the philosophy and practice of Yoga to the System was truly substantial.

Yoga to a great extent defined the vocabulary of the System and the structure of its development and exposition.

Yoga provided the System with multiple 'training and drill' exercises for the actor's internal and external technique. Perfection of a significant number of elements of the creative sense of self in the Stanislavsky System up to the present has been accomplished through methods going back to the centuries-old yogic tradition.

Yoga helped to formulate the core concept of the System about the unconscious and its division into the subconscious and the superconscious. 'The subconscious creative work of nature through the conscious psycho-technique of the actor.'[286]

Yoga suggested *practical ways* of realizing the fundamental principle of the System: from the conscious to the unconscious. As opposed to Western mentality, contrasting the body and the conscious, Yoga offered Stanislavsky an integral, holistic view of man. Stanislavsky used Yoga exercises to help actors cross borders created by the materiality of the body, and, using superior levels of the creative conscious, to break through to the transcendental, the Supreme.

Yoga provided Stanislavsky with a model which answered the questions of the System about the interrelations of the body and the spirit to a greater extent than the psychology of his time.

Yoga paved the way for the synthesizing discoveries of Stanislavsky in his late period: the concept of the indissolubility of the psychophysical existence of man; the Method of Action Analysis; and the technique of etudes in which the System

[286] Stanislavskii, *Ss* 9, II (1989), 61.

finally appeared as a complete approach to an actor's creative work involving all aspects of his apparatus – the conscious, the body, and the spirit.

Today, having lived through the historically conditioned period of the concealment of the yogic component of the System and rejecting the exaggeration of its significance (under the influence of Perestroika), we can carefully analyze the mutual intersections of Yoga teaching and the System. The practice of modern theatre life itself demands that we realize and consider Yoga as one of the sources of Stanislavsky's methodology. The present work proposes only the direction of such analysis and is among the first steps on that path.

It goes without saying that future research will give us many intriguing surprises. The meeting with Edward Gordon Craig and Isadora Duncan made Stanislavsky note:

> I understood that in different parts of the world, on account of conditions unknown to us, different people, in different fields, coming from different directions, are searching in art for the same recurrent, naturally born creative principles. When they meet, they are struck by the community and kinship of their ideas.[287]

We can only imagine how surprised Stanislavsky himself would be to find out that the books, brought to his attention in France by the medical student of a Buryat Buddhist physician from Saint Petersburg and containing an account of the teaching of ancient Indian yogis, were written by an American author from Chicago. Likewise, he would be astounded that his own books about the System published in Moscow and New York would so forcefully inspire as well as cause such fiery debate throughout the whole theatrical world of America; and that almost a hundred years later theatre scholars and practitioners on both sides of the ocean would engage in a parallel reading of Ramacharaka and Stanislavsky, surprised at their anticipation of the discoveries of contemporary neurobiology.

---

[287] Stanislavskii, *Ss* 9, I (1988), 413.

Indeed, this curious circulation of ideas looks like a chapter from a detective novel and is definitely not deprived of expressive theatricality. It seems that Yoga and Theatre met completely by chance, but we might say this meeting was fated to happen. And though it took place at the very beginning of the twentieth century, the interaction of the two happily continues. Today the union of Yoga and the Stanislavsky System determines – obviously or invisibly – contemporary actor training and theatre practice both in Russia and throughout the world.

Bibliography

ABALKIN, Nikolai A., *Sistema Stanislavskogo i sovetskii teatr*, 2nd edn (Moscow: Iskusstvo, 1954)

ALBANESE, Catherine, *A Republic of Mind and Spirit* (New Haven: Yale University Press, 2007)

ANTAROVA, Koncordia E., *Besedy K. S. Stanislavskogo v studii Bolshogo teatra v 1918-1922 gg* (Moscow: Iskusstvo, 1952)

BASHINDZHAGIAN, Natella Z., *Kontury biografii: Ezhi Grotovskii. Ot Bednogo teatra k Iskusstvu-provodniku* (Moscow: Akter. Regisser. Teatr, 2003)

BOLESLAVSKY, Richard, *Lances Down* (New York: Garden City, 1932)

CARNICKE, Sharon Marie, *Stanislavsky in Focus* (The Netherlands: Harwood Academic Publishers, 1998), 138–145

CARNICKE, Sharon Marie, *Stanislavsky in Focus: An Acting Master for the Twenty-First Century*, 2nd edn (London and New York: Routledge, 2009)

CHEKHOV, Mikhail A., *Literaturnoe nasledie v 2 t.*, 2nd edn (Moscow: Iskusstvo, 1995)

CHERNAIA, Elena I., *Kurs treninga fonatsionnogo dykhaniia i fonatsii na osnove uprazhnenii Vostoka* (Saint Petersburg: SPbGATI, 1997)

— *Vospitanie fonatsionnogo dykhaniia s ispolzovaniem printsipov dykhatelnoi gimnastiki 'iogi'* (Moscow: Granitsa, 2009)

DAMASIO, Antonio, *The Feeling of What Happens: Body and Emotion in the Making of Consciousness* (New York: Penguin, 1999)

De MICHELIS, Elizabeth, 'Modern Yoga: History and Forms' in *Yoga in the Modern World: Contemporary Perspectives*, ed. by Mark Singleton and Jean Byrne (Oxon: Routledge, 2008)

DIKII, Alexei D., *Povest o teatralnoi iunosti* (Moscow: Iskusstvo, 1957)

DODIN, Lev A., 'Chelovek – sushchestvo tragicheskoe, i emu neobxodimo tragicheskoe iskusstvo: Interviu Iu. Kovalenko', *Izvestiya*, 6 May 1997

DYBOVSKII, Vladimir V., 'V plenu predlagaemykh obstoiatelstv', *Minuvshee: istoricheskii almanakh*, X, 243–320 (Moscow and Saint Petersburg: Atheneum-Feniks, 1992)

ELLENBERGER, Henri, *The Discovery of the Unconscious* (New York: Basic Books, 1970)

FOVITZKY, A. L., *The Moscow Art Theatre and Its Distinguishing Characteristics* (New York: Chernoff Publishing Co., 1923)

GALENDEEV, Valerii N., *Uchenie K. S. Stanislavskogo o stsenicheskom slove* (Leningrad: LGITMiK, 1990)

GIATSINTOVA, Sofia V., *S pamatiu naedine*, 2nd edn (Moscow: Iskusstvo, 1989)

GIPPIUS, Sergei V., *Gimnastika chuvstv. Trenning tvorcheskoi psikhotekhniki* (Moscow and Leningrad: Iskusstvo, 1967)

— *Trenning razvitiia kreativnosti. Gimnastika chuvstv* (Saint Petersburg: Rech, 2001)

GRACHEVA, Larisa V., 'Psikhotekhnika aktera v processe obucheniia: teoriia i praktika' (dissertation for the D.Sc. degree in Theatre Studies, Saint Petersburg State Theatre Arts Academy, 2005)

GORDON, Mel, *The Stanislavsky Technique: Russia* (New York: Applause Theatre Book Publishers, 1987)

— *Stanislavsky in America: An Actor's Workbook* (London and New York: Routledge, 2010)

GRAY, Paul, 'The Reality of Doing: Interviews with Vera Soloviova, Stella Adler, and Sanford Meisner', in *Stanislavski and America*, ed. by Erika Munk (New York: Hill and Wang, 1964), 201–18

GREKOVA, Tatiana I., 'Tibetskaia medetsina v Rossii', *Nauka i religiia*, 8 (1988), 10–15

GROTOWSKI, Jerzy, *Towards a Poor Theatre* (New York: Simon and Schuster, 1968)

— *Ot bednogo teatra k iskusstvu-provodniku*, trans. by N. Z. Bashindzhagian (Moscow: ART, 2003)

HIRSCH, Foster, *A Method to their Madness: The History of the Actors Studio*, 2nd edn (Cambridge MA: Da Capo, 2002)

IVANOV, Vladislav V., 'Introduction to "Lektsii Rudolfa Shtainera o dramaticheskom iskusstve v izlozhenii Mikhaila Chekhova. Pisma aktera k V. A. Gromovu"', *Mnemozina: Dokumenty i fakty iz istorii otechestvennogo teatra XX veka: Istoricheskii almanakh*, II, ed. by V. V. Ivanov (Moscow: Editorial URSS, 2006), 85–91

KAPSALI, Maria, 'The Use of Yoga in Actor Training and Theatre Making' (unpublished Ph.D. dissertation in Performance Practice [Drama], University of Exeter, 2010)

— '"I don't attack it but it's not for actors": The Use of Yoga by Jerzy Grotowski', *Theatre, Dance and Performance Training*, 1 (2) (2010), 185–98

— 'Towards a Body-Mind Spirituality: The Practice of Yoga and the Case of Air', *Journal of Dance and Somatic Practices*, 1 (4) (2012), 109–24

— 'The Presence of Yoga in Stanislavski's Work', *Stanislavski Studies*, 3 (2013), 139–50 <http://stanislavskistudies.org>

— 'Rethinking Actor Training: Training Body, Mind and… Ideological Awareness', *Theatre Dance and Performance Training*, 4 (1) (2013), 73–86

— 'The "Ancient" Body of Modern Yoga: The influence of Ramanuja on Iyengar Yoga and the use of Iyengar Yoga in Actor Training', *Studies in South Asian Film and Media*, 4 (2) (2013), 11–23

KOSTIUCHENKO, Vladislav S., *Vivekananda* (Moscow: Misl, 1977)

KRISTI, Grigorii V., 'Kniga K. S. Stanislavskogo "Rabota aktera nad soboi"' in Stanislavskii, Konstantin Sergeevich, *Sobranie sochinenii v 8 t.*, II (Moscow: Iskusstvo, 1954–1961), p. xviii

LARIONOV, Mikhail F., *Luchism* (Moscow: K. and K.,1913)

LOBANOVA, Olga G., *Pravilnoe dykhanie Olgi Lobanovoi: Pervaia rossiiskaia dykhatelnaia praktika* (Saint Petersburg: Nevskii Prospekt, 2005)

— *Dyshite pravilno: Uchenie indiiskikh iogov o dykhanii, izmenennoe Zapadom. Amerikanskaia metoda Koflera*, 2nd edn (Moscow: Librokom, 2012)

MANDERINO, Ned, *Stanislavski's Fourth Level: A Super-conscious Approach to Acting* (Los Angeles: Manderino Books, 2001)

MCCANNON, John, 'In Search of Primeval Russia: Stylistic Evolution in the Landscapes of Nicholas Roerich, 1897–1914', *Cultural Geographies*, 7 (3) (2000), 271–97

MCCARTNEY, James, *Philosophy and Practice of Yoga* (Romford: L.N. Fowler and Co, 1978)

MEYERHOLD, Vsevolod E., *Stati, pisma, rechi, besedy*, 2 vols (Moscow: Iskusstvo, 1968)

OSIŃSKI, Zbigniew, *Jerzy Grotowski's Journeys to the East* (Holstebro, Malta, Wrocław, London and New York: Icarus and Routledge, 2014)

POLIAKOVA, Elena I., *Stanislavskii* (Moscow: Iskusstvo, 1977)

— *Teatr Sulerzhitskogo: Etika. Estetika. Rezhissura* (Moscow: Agraf, 2006)

RAMACHARAKA, *Hatha Yoga; or, The Yogi Philosophy of Physical Well-Being* (Chicago: Yogi Publication Society, 1904); PDF file available at https://archive.org/details/hathayoga00rama

— *A Series of Lessons in Raja Yoga* (Chicago: Yogi Publication Society, 1906); PDF file available at https://archive.org/details/seriesoflessonsi00rama

RADISCHEVA, Olga A., *Stanislavskii i Nemirovich-Danchenko: Istoriia teatralnykh otnoshenii, 1917-1938* (Moscow: Akter. Regisser. Teatr, 1999)

RIBOT, Théodule, *Psikhologiia vnimaniia* (Saint Petersburg: F. Pavlenkov, 1897)

ROACH, Joseph, *The Player's Passion* (Newark: University of Delaware Press, 1985)

RUMIANTSEV, Pavel I., *Stanislavskii i opera* (Moscow: Iskusstvo, 1969)

SCHECHNER, Richard, 'Exoduction', *The Grotowski Sourcebook*, ed. by Liza Wolford and Richard Schechner (London: Routledge, 1997), 462–94

SHVERUBOVICH, Vadim V., *O liudiakh, o teatre i o sebe* (Moscow: Iskusstvo, 1976)

SILANTEVA, Irina I. and Klimenko Yurii G., *Akter i ego Alter Ego* (Moscow: Graal, 2000)

SIMONOV, Pavel V., *Metod K. S. Stanislavskogo i fiziologiia emotsii* (Moscow: Izd. AN SSSR, 1962)

— 'Soznanie, podsoznanie, sverkhsoznanie', *Nauka*, 12 (1975), 45–51

— 'Kategoriia soznaniia, podsoznaniia i sverkhsoznaniia v tvorcheskoi sisteme K. S. Stanislavskogo' in *Bessoznatelnoe. Priroda. Funktsii. Metody Issledovanii*, II (Tbilisi: Metsniereba, 1978), 518–27

— '"Sverkhsoznanie" i "sverkhzadacha"' in *Stanislavskii v meniaiushchemsia mire* (Moscow: Blagotvoritelnyi fond K. S. Stanislavskogo, 1994), 201–04

SMELIANSKY, Anatoly M., 'Professiia – artist' in Konstantin Stanislavskii, *Sobranie sochinenii v 9 t.*, II (Moscow: Iskusstvo, 1989), 5–38

STANISLAVSKI, Constantin, *An Actor Prepares*, trans. by Elizabeth Reynolds Hapgood (New York: Theatre Arts Books, 1936)

— *Building a Character*, trans. by Elizabeth Reynolds Hapgood (New York: Theatre Arts Books, 1949)

— *Creating a Role*, trans. by Elizabeth Reynolds Hapgood (New York: Theatre Arts Books, 1961)

STANISLAVSKI, Konstantin, *An Actor's Work*, trans. by Jean Benedetti (London and New York: Routledge, 2008)

— *An Actor's Work on a Role*, trans. by Jean Benedetti (London and New York: Routledge, 2010)

STANISLAVSKII, Konstantin Sergeevich, *Sobranie sochi-nenii v 8 t.* (Moscow: Iskusstvo: 1954–1961)

— *Sobranie sochinenii v 9 t.* (Moscow: Iskusstvo, 1988–1999)

— *Iz zapisnykh knizhek*, 2 vols (Moscow: VTO, 1986)

— *Stanislavskii repetiruet. Zapisi i stenogrammy repetitsii*, ed. by I. N. Vinogradskaia (Moscow: STD RSFSR, 1987)

STRASBERG, Lee, 'Notes from the Laboratory Theatre' in the file 'Lab Theatre', Archive of the Lee Strasberg Theatre and Film Institute (New York, 1924–25)

SULLIVAN, John, 'Stanislavski and Freud' in *Stanislavski and America*, ed. by Erika Munk (New York: Hill and Wang, 1966), 88–109

SUKHANOV, Sergei L., 'Podsoznanie i ego patologiia', *Voprosy filosofii i psikhologii*, 26 (128) (1915), 362–77

SUSHKEVICH, Boris M., *Sem momentov raboty nad roliu* (Leningrad: Izd. Gos. Akadem. Teatra dramy, 1933)

TAGORE, Rabindranath, *Sādhanā* (New York: Doubleday, 2004)

TCHERKASSKI, Sergei D., *Valentin Smyshliaev – akter, rezhisser, pedagog* (Saint Petersburg: SPbGATI, 2004)

— 'Stanislavskii i ioga: opyt parallelnogo chteniia', *Voprosy teatra; Proscaenium*, 3–4 (2009), 282–300

— 'Iogicheskie element sistemy Stanislavskogo', *Voprosy teatra; Proscaenium*, 1–2 (2010), 252–70

— 'The Directing and Teaching of Richard Boleslavsky and Lee Strasberg as an Experiment in the Stanislavsky System's Development' (dissertation for the D.Sc. degree in Theatre Studies, Saint Petersburg State Theatre Arts Academy, 2012)

TCHERKASSKI, Sergei, 'Fundamentals of the Stanislavski System and Yoga Philosophy and Practice, Part 1', *Stanislavski Studies*, 1 (2012), 1–18 <http://stanislavskistudies. org/category/issues/issue-1/>

— 'Fundamentals of the Stanislavski System and Yoga Philosophy and Practice, Part 2', *Stanislavski Studies*, 2 (2013), 190–236 <http://stanislavskistudies.org>

— 'The System Becomes the Method: Stanislavsky – Boleslavsky – Strasberg', *Stanislavski Studies*, 3 (2013), 92–138 <http://stanislavskistudies.org>

TIULIAEV, Semen I., 'Konkordiia Antarova: M. Strizhenova, iz vospominanii', *Sait Lotosa. Entsiklopediia sovremennoi ezoteriki* <http://ariom.ru/wiki/KonkordijaAntarova>

VAKHTANGOV, Evgenii, *Evgenii Vakhtangov. Dokumenty i svidetelstva*, 2 vol., ed. by V. V. Ivanovov (Moscow: Indrik, 2011)

VAKHTANGOV, Evgenii, *Sbornik* (Moscow: VTO, 1984)

VINOGRADSKAIA, Irina N., *Zhizn i tvorchestvo K. S. Stanislavskogo: Letopis v 4 t.* (Moscow: MXT, 2003)

WEGNER, William H., 'The Creative Circle: Stanislavski and Yoga', *Educational Theatre Journal*, 28 (1) (1976), 85–89

WHITE, Andrew, 'Stanislavsky and Ramacharaka: The Influence of Yoga and Turn-of-the-Century Occultism on the System', *Theater Survey*, 47 (1) (2006), 73–92

— 'Stanislavsky and Ramacharaka: The Impact of Yoga and the Occult Revival of the System' in *The Routledge Companion to Stanislavsky*, ed. by R. Andrew White (London and New York: Routledge, 2014), 287–304

WHYMAN, Rose, *The Stanislavsky System of Acting: Legacy and Influence in Modern Performance* (Cambridge: Cambridge University Press, 2008)

YOGANANDA, Paramahansa, *Autobiography of a Yogi* (Los Angeles: Self-Realization Fellowship, 1946)

Index